Law and Ethics
for Advanced
Practice Nursing

Diane Kjervik, JD, MSN, RN, FAAN, is Professor and Chair, School of Nursing, of the University of North Carolina–Chapel Hill. She received a BSN from the University of Wisconsin–Madison, an MS in Psychiatric Nursing from the University of California at San Francisco, and a JD from William Mitchell College of Law, St. Paul, Minnesota. She served as the Director of the Carolina Women's Center and as President of the American Association of Nurse Attorneys (TAANA). She is also a member of numerous organizations, such as the American Bar Association and the American Nurses Association. In both 1998 and 2004, she received the TAANA Outstanding Advocate Award and, in 2006, she received the prestigious Mary Turner Lane Award from the Association of Women Faculty and Professionals at UNC–Chapel Hill for her work on behalf of women. She is a peer reviewer for many journals, and has reviewed grants for federal agencies, including the National Library of Medicine, the Bureau of Health Professions in Rockville, Maryland, and the Advisory Council for the National Center for Nursing Research at the National Institutes of Health. She also served as Chair of the Committee on Standards for Legal Content in Nursing Education of TAANA, and as Director of Governmental Relations and Associate Director of Research for the American Association of Colleges of Nursing. Professor Kjervik has served as Editor-in-Chief of the *Journal of Nursing Law* for the past 16 years; is the author of numerous articles, chapters, and books; and is a frequent speaker on topics dealing with the legal rights and ethical responsibilities of health professionals.

Edith Ann Brous, MS, MPH, JD, RN, received her BSN from Wayne State University in 1978, her MS from Columbia University College of Nursing and MPH from Columbia University School of Public Health in 1995, and her JD from Fordham University School of Law in 1999. She is currently in private practice as a nurse attorney who specializes in medical malpractice, professional licensure defense, and nursing advocacy legislation. She held previous positions at Martin, Clearwater and Bell, LLP; DLA Piper; and Garson, Gerspach, DeCorato, and Cohen, LLP. Prior to her practice of law, she was the Assistant Director of Nursing for Emergency and Hyperbaric Services at Cabrini Medical Center in New York City. She is a contributing editor on legal issues for the *American Journal of Nursing* and has published extensively in the nursing literature on law and law-related issues. Ms. Brous is adjunct faculty at several universities and lectures throughout the country on legal aspects of nursing practice. She is a member of many Bar associations and professional nursing organizations and is the current President-Elect of The American Association of Nurse Attorneys.

Law and Ethics
for Advanced
Practice Nursing

DIANE KJERVIK, JD, MSN, RN, FAAN
EDITH ANN BROUS, MS, MPH, JD, RN

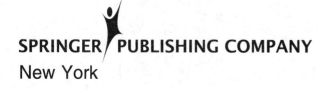

SPRINGER PUBLISHING COMPANY
New York

Springer Publishing Company, LLC
11 West 42nd Street
New York, NY 10036
www.springerpub.com

Acquisitions Editor: Allan Graubard
Project Editor: Peter Rocheleau
Project Manager: Pamela Lankas
Cover Design: Steve Pisano
Composition: International Graphic Services

ISBN: 978-0-8261-1458-7
Ebook ISBN: 978-0-8261-1459-4

10 11 12 13/ 5 4 3 2 1

The author and the publisher of this Work have made every effort to use sources believed to be reliable to provide information that is accurate and compatible with the standards generally accepted at the time of publication. Because medical science is continually advancing, our knowledge base continues to expand. Therefore, as new information becomes available, changes in procedures become necessary. We recommend that the reader always consult current research and specific institutional policies before performing any clinical procedure. The author and publisher shall not be liable for any special, consequential, or exemplary damages resulting, in whole or in part, from the readers' use of, or reliance on, the information contained in this book. The publisher has no responsibility for the persistence or accuracy of URLs for external or third-party Internet Web sites referred to in this publication and does not guarantee that any content on such Web sites is, or will remain, accurate or appropriate.

Library of Congress Cataloging-in-Publication Data

Kjervik, Diane K., 1945-
Law and ethics for advanced practice nursing / Diane Kjervik, Edith Ann Brous.
    p. ; cm.
  Includes bibliographical references and index.
  ISBN 978-0-8261-1458-7--ISBN 978-0-8261-1459-4 (e-book)
   1. Nurse practitioners—Legal status, laws, etc.—United States. 2. Nursing—Law and legislation—United States. 3. Nursing ethics—United States. 4. Nursing—Practice—United States. 5. Nursing—Law and legislation. I. Brous, Edith Ann. II. Title.
  [DNLM: 1. Advanced Practice Nursing—legislation & jurisprudence—United States. 2. Advanced Practice Nursing—ethics—United States. WY 33 AA1 K62L 2010]
  KF2915.N8K54 2010
  344.7304'14—dc22
                                                2010018394

Printed in the United States of America by Bang Printing

We lovingly dedicate this book to our fathers
Dr. Abner R. Kjervik and Hugh B. Brous, Jr.
for their inspiration and a lifetime of guidance

Contents

Contributors

Debra J. Barksdale, PhD, FNP-BC, ANP-BC, CNE, FAANP, is an Associate Professor at the University of North Carolina at Chapel Hill (UNC-CH) School of Nursing. She is certified as both a family and an adult nurse practitioner. She is also a certified nurse educator and is a Fellow of the American Academy of Nurse Practitioners. She is nationally known for work with nurse practitioner education and diversity and was recently appointed to the Nursing Education Advisory Council of the National League for Nursing. She chairs the Master's Executive Committee; co-chairs the Graduate Faculty Committee; and is a member of the Faculty Development Committee, the Ethnic Minority Visiting Scholars Task Force, and the Faculty Executive Committee in the SON. She is currently a leader in efforts to establish a Doctor of Nursing Practice Program at UNC-CH. She was coordinator of the FNP Program at UNC-CH for 4 years. She was also a Department of Health and Human Services (DHHS) Primary Health Care Policy Fellow and a member of the Board of Directors of the prestigious National Organization of Nurse Practitioner Faculty (NONPF). Additionally, Dr. Barksdale is a researcher with an NIH-funded grant focusing on stress and cardiovascular responses in African Americans. She currently practices at the Robert Nixon Clinic in Chapel Hill and has over 20 years of NP experience in urgent care, primary care, home care, and care of the underserved. Dr. Barksdale is a practitioner, educator, researcher, administrator, and advocate.

Gina Raineri Bernain, JD, RN, is currently an Assistant Professor in the Bioethics Department of the School of Medicine at the Universidad de Chile where she is also the Executive Secretary of the Interfaculty Program of the Medicine and Law Schools. She is a member of the Colegio de Abogados de Chile, as well as the Ethics Committee of the Hospital Luis Calvo Mackenna, and the Hospital Exequiel González Cortes, both located in Santiago, Chile.

Arlene M Davis, RN, JD, is Associate Professor of Social Medicine at the UNC-Chapel Hill School of Medicine and Adjunct Associate Professor at the UNC School of Law. Professor Davis teaches graduate students in medicine, nursing, and law on various bioethics and health law topics. The majority of her research ethics teaching and scholarship is conducted as an investigator in the UNC Center for Genomics and Society and as core ethics faculty for the North Carolina Translational Research and Clinical Sciences Institute. Her clinical ethics work centers on patient care; she serves as Director of Clinical Ethics Consultation and Education for UNC Healthcare and its hospital ethics committee. Professor Davis is also a Fellow at the Parr Center for Bioethics at UNC and a long-standing institutional review board (IRB) member at Research Triangle Institute International. She is licensed to practice law in North Carolina.

Foreword

The expertise of advanced practice nurses (APNs) has expanded the standards of care beyond basic nursing care. With increased expertise, additional benefits and obligations are important for APNs to be aware of as they provide both legal and ethical care. *Law and Ethics for Advanced Practice Nursing* provides a comprehensive overview, including the details needed to understand the obligations and rights for APN practice. The authors are experts in understanding the legal and ethical dimensions of advanced practice nursing, and they employed extensive legal research to examine the opportunities and expectations of APNs.

In chapter 1, the history of the changes that have led from limited autonomy to increasing levels of responsibility for APNs is discussed. Legal cases that give insight into successful defenses to malpractice cases involving statutes of limitation, practice standards, and causal connections between patient injuries and APN interventions are presented. These cases demonstrate for the APN how the law evaluates APN liability. Cases that discuss intentional misrepresentation of professional credentials and improper use of controlled substances also provide important lessons for APNs. Legal cases involving the APN's professional practice, such as third-party reimbursement and the APN's expertise to testify in civil and criminal cases, clarify both rights and responsibilities for APN practice. Patient privacy rights, antitrust violations, slander, and intentional infliction of emotional distress as causes of action are also discussed in cases addressing hospital and prescriptive authority privileges. The law applying to the APN's practice is constantly evolving through the findings and holdings of legal cases. The lessons learned through the experiences of APNs in the cases discussed in chapter 1 are important for preventive risk management in the APN's practice. The relationship between APNs and physicians, including noncompete covenants, is also an important historical perspective in this chapter.

Chapter 2 discusses the interface of nursing law and ethics. Ethical dilemmas present situations that do not always have the same outcomes, because not all people choose to live or die in the same way. The solutions to these issues are gray areas where there are no right or wrong answers, and these are decisions that should be made by those who have the right to make an informed decision. When members of a society cannot agree on how serious ethical dilemmas should be decided, and who has the right to make the decision, the issue often becomes a legal consideration. Courts then decide how a resolution must be reached. The APN's role as the patient advocate, and an advocate for the APN's practice, is considered in this challenging chapter.

Chapter 3 informs the readers about policy changes affecting APN practice. Educational, licensure, certification, and accreditation requirements nationally are all policy decisions that affect the rights of APNs to practice their profession as partners with physicians and other providers. APNs need to stay involved in the process of policy development in order to protect their right to legally provide care based upon their skills, efforts, and responsibilities.

Fair compensation for APN services is also an important policy issue discussed in this chapter. Strategies for building consensus within the profession, as well as support from consumers, employers, and co-workers, are vital in order to enable policy development that will allow APNs to provide high quality and affordable care.

Chapter 4 provides the information needed to understand malpractice, or nursing negligence. The facts needed to understand the APN's responsibilities as the patient's advocate and caregiver are discussed in a clear and understandable way that displaces unnecessary fears of malpractice. Statistics on actual malpractice actions against APNs are provided. Insurance issues and reductions in medical errors are discussed as supportive information for the APN's risk-management planning. Discussion of patient perceptions and why patients sue are especially helpful in assisting APNs to minimize their malpractice risks.

Chapter 5 is especially important to APNs, as the issues of labor and employment become more individualized through the expertise and licensure opportunities of the APN. The different employment relationships available to APNs are discussed in clear and helpful terms. Regulations, rights, and responsibilities based on worker classifications are important to understand when deciding whether to set up a private practice or to accept employment from a physician group or hospital. Recommendations on purchasing professional liability insurance, even when choosing to be employed by another, are shared in this helpful chapter.

Chapter 6 clarifies the foundations of licensure and regulations through an interesting discussion of the history of how the profession of nursing evolved. The development of Nurse Practice Acts, and finally, the expanded APN role, as well as the role of State Boards of Nursing, are described in this chapter. Licensure is a privilege that APNs must earn. Every state has its individual requirements that must be understood by APNs who practice and are licensed in multiple states. State Boards of Nursing have been delegated the legal authority to ensure compliance with the nursing standards imposed by their state to safeguard the public, as well as the APN's right to practice. The moral character of the APN may also become a concern of the State Board of Nursing if a complaint is made against the APN. The information shared in this chapter will assist the reader in understanding the system within which APNs work.

Chapter 7, Nursing and Law Pedagogy for APNs, provides an interesting and important opportunity for APNs to learn how to use the connection between law and nursing theory to become policy advocates for patients, families, and communities. Understanding this connection provides the conceptual framework for testing legal, ethical, and nursing phenomena together. Evidence-based information provides a powerful tool for change in building interdisciplinary strength. The future power of the APN's practice is obvious from the information provided in this chapter, based upon the author's experience and expertise.

Chapter 8 brings the reader to the global issues of international law and nursing. The nursing shortage that extended throughout the 1990s was a global experience. The impact of the shortage was, however, felt differently across the world, depending on the economic resources of the country. Statistics shared in this chapter describe the accelerated migration of nurses from economically deprived countries to resource-rich countries. The ethics of a global nursing society with the goal of global public health is the message of this important final chapter of the book.

The eight chapters in this book are interesting and offer easy reading. The complex topics discussed are expertly shared through the knowledge, skill, and understanding of the authors, who are both nurses and attorneys. The needs of APN practitioners have been thoughtfully evaluated and presented in this comprehensive text.

Penny Brooke, APRN, JD
Professor and Coordinator of Service-Learning
College of Nursing
University of Utah

Preface

What were the visionaries in nursing seeing as they imagined advanced practice in nursing? A portion of their story involved the law, which, as they found it, stood in the way of their expanded practice. In 1979, Shirley Berglund, a nurse practitioner in St. Paul, Minnesota, became the first nurse practitioner in that state to incorporate her business, establish her office, and "hang out her shingle." She maintained an active practice until 1991, when she closed her office and sold the building. She led the way in Minnesota, as others did across the country, to pave the way for advanced practice nurses (APNs) who wanted to conduct independent businesses in collaboration with other health providers. Nursing, in their view, was its own professional discipline, not a part of medicine, pharmacy, public health, or social work. Rather, it could and indeed would stand on its own in service to consumers who sought nursing expertise. This book constitutes a tribute to the APNs, such as Shirley Berglund, who fought, suffered, endured, and succeeded in their challenge to the status quo.

With its emphasis on the legal tools used by APN pioneers and the ethical foundations on which they built their practices, this book provides a unique examination of historical and recent legal challenges these nurses faced. Some barriers were overcome, and some yet remain. However, the momentum for advanced practice won't be slowed in the environment of increased cost constraints and consumer demand for access to high-quality care. APNs are charting their course, and the law can help or hinder these efforts, depending on the degree of engagement and sophistication APNs have about legal process and decisions. This book provides insights to guide nurses and nursing leaders as they develop their strategies for change.

Law as a source of power guided by ethics as a source of philosophical sophistication provides the backbone of a concerted strategy for continuing development of the nursing profession. Conflicting ethical obligations exist, however, challenging the APN's sense of integrity. This book presents approaches to understanding and resolving several of these ethical conflicts. Nursing research, theory, and knowledge cannot shine on their own without corresponding policies that are open to these insights. Evidence created by nursing researchers and scholars is best created with attention paid to legal and ethical phenomena. Thus, this book is intended for APNs in practice, nursing educators teaching in APN programs, and for basic and applied nursing researchers who are studying phenomena of concern to APNs. The book will also be a resource for lawyers and ethicists who work with or on behalf of APNs.

From a practical standpoint, the book includes cases that make legal precedent in specific jurisdictions, and as such, are limited to that jurisdiction. However, courts reason by analogy, and although one state's decisions are not binding on another state, each court may use the arguments from another judge or jurisdiction to support its new ruling. Likewise, some cases presented here center on staff nurses, physicians, or other health providers, and not on APNs. However, the precedent set is likely to be followed by the court when faced with a similar case involving an APN. The cases have been selected to illustrate legal principles and the manner in which the courts analyze them, not to highlight their outcomes. Information regarding the dispute's final resolution is actually irrelevant, and may not be available or discussed in cases that were remanded back to the trial level, because it is generally only the appeals court that publishes decisions and opinions. Also, areas of law such as malpractice, contract, and civil rights often intersect. The cases presented here will highlight one area of law, but mention may be made of other, related areas. Important to note is that law that is settled in a jurisdiction is often based on cases that are from years before. Thus, cases cited in this book will, at times, be from older case precedents that have not been overturned. The legal world refers to those cases as still representing "good law." Additionally, some older cases were selected because they established or changed the law and provide historical perspective.

From a linguistic standpoint, the language of law includes words such as "test" and "theory" that are used differently from the way they are used in health care. A legal test is a set of criteria to help the court decide whether a certain requirement is met. A legal theory is an area of law such as negligence or contract, upon which the parties to litigation rest their complaint against the other party. And, of course, there are obvious differences in use of language, such as "labor law," which has to do with union relationships and not obstetrical experience. Throughout the book, the authors define terminology specific to the legal decisions they address, and in this way, they serve as translators of legal language for the health care audience.

We present this knowledge with the hope that APNs and those who work with and for them will find these insights and suggestions of help as they build and refine educational, research, and practice programs. We are grateful to our consultants, who assisted us as we developed the book. And we offer a special thanks to our publisher, who envisioned the need for this book and sought our expertise to create this publication.

Diane Kjervik
Edie Brous

Law and Ethics for Advanced Practice Nursing

1

Law as a Partner in the Expansion of Advanced Practice Nursing Roles

DIANE KJERVIK

The question, then, must lie not with the existence of nursing authority, but with people's recognition of that authority.

—*E. Baer*

The tale of the evolution of advanced practice nursing (APN) begins with the roles that nurses played in hospitals and their wish to find independence outside the hospital. The law represents a form of power that assisted nurses to move beyond their traditional roles to grasp the ones they hoped to assume over time. Ellen Baer describes the source of this process as nursing's "growing militancy in its refusal to be dominated by medicine" (Baer, 1993, p. 111). Ethics provided the expression of values in support of nurses' empowerment, namely, autonomy in practice, beneficence and care-based ethic in doing what is best for patients, and justice (fair treatment of all providers and patients). This chapter will examine exemplary ethically embedded legal cases that, taken together, frame pivotal moments in the history of advanced practice nurses (APNs) from the 1950s through the 1980s.

The earliest nurse practitioner (NP) program, crafted in 1965 by Loretta Ford and Henry Silver in response to a shortage of primary care physicians, emphasized the primary care model of health promotion and disease prevention (McGivern, 1993). As health care reform efforts arose, the need for more primary care providers intensified (Inglis &

1

Kjervik, 1993). Interestingly, many of the early legal cases involving APNs centered on nurse anesthetists and other APNs working in acute care settings.

The cases are divided into two categories: (a) those addressing expanded roles and privileges, such as intentional and unintentional actions (standard of care), expertise and courtroom testimony, and hospital and prescriptive privileges; and (b) those stemming from relationships between APNs and physicians, such as antitrust and insurance, noncompete clauses, and supervision by MDs. Both expanding scopes of practice and substandard levels of performance, as discussed by Bartter (2001), comprise the content of these cases. The results of legal research of cases covered here exemplify controversies that have been taken to court for resolution. Because many cases are settled prior to trial, only the published court decisions resulting in precedents in those jurisdictions are presented here. Some of the cases are transferred back (remanded) to a lower court for final action. Litigants may then settle the case without benefit of trial or further written opinion. Similarly, no written record of trial court opinions on the state level exists, so final disposition of these cases remains unknown. The cases are organized chronologically to highlight the changes in the legal view of APNs over time.

ROLES AND PRIVILEGES

Standard of Care

The legal standard of care for a health professional sets the expected performance of a nurse, and evolves over time as clinical practice changes and nursing roles expand. Each state sets its own standard of care, and must be researched thoroughly for precedent. The first set of cases addresses negligence, the failure to meet the standard of care that results in injury to a patient.

Unintentional Acts (Negligence)

In 1954, a case was brought against a hospital and an MD, which also involved the actions of a nurse anesthetist, for negligent actions during an attempted tonsillectomy. The nurse anesthetist at the hospital intubated the patient so that the tube went to the stomach, rather than the lungs, resulting in painful abdominal distention after the intubation. She was found negligent under *respondeat superior*, the principle that the employer is responsible for negligent acts of the employee. The surgeon was found not to be responsible for the acts of the nurse anesthetist. The physician, the surgeon in this situation, was an eye, ear, nose, and throat specialist who did not supervise or have control over the nurse anesthetist. She was an employee of the hospital, and her testimony at trial specified that she received no supervision from the surgeon. On appeal, the Supreme Court of Washington affirmed the judgment of the trial court (*Kemalyan v. Henderson*, 1954).

In contrast, a case involving the administration of penicillin to a patient who was allergic to it resulted in a different legal outcome in Pennsylvania. As a result of the administration of penicillin to the patient, a severe allergic reaction and cardiovascular accident occurred. The *respondeat superior* doctrine was used to find that an MD was responsible for the acts of a nurse anesthetist and a resident who failed to act on information they had about a surgical patient's allergy to penicillin (*Yorston v. Pennell*, 1959).

In 1964, a patient who suffered impaired functionality of her arm following gynecological surgery alleged that the Certified Registered Nurse Anesthetist (CRNA) who administered sodium pentothal punctured a vein, and as a result, the muscle tissue near the site was damaged. In finding for the CRNA, a federal District Court in Michigan found no malpractice, and concluded that the CRNA and the surgeon followed customary practice in the administration of sodium pentothal, with its concomitant risks and lack of direct supervision of the CRNA by the surgeon. The court strongly stated that, "a treating physician, surgeon, or nurse-anesthetist is not a warrantor in performing medical or surgical services. They are responsible in damages for unfortunate results when, and only when, it is shown that they have departed from the standard in the community of treatment and care by skilled doctors and nurses" (*Gore v. United States*, 1964, p. 549). The court also noted that the Michigan nurse practice act changed in 1952 from the expectation that an MD supervise and direct RNs to the expectation the RNs carry out treatments as prescribed by a physician.

In South Dakota in 1975, a nurse anesthetist chose penthrane, a halogenated anesthetic, for a cholecystectomy. The physician recalled suggesting that she not use a halogenated anesthetic, but the nurse anesthetist had no such recollection. A few days after the surgery, the patient died of liver failure, and this wrongful death legal action was instituted by the patient's husband. The defendants won in the trial court, but on appeal, the question of the type of witness needed in a malpractice case against a nurse anesthetist, a physician, and a hospital was raised. During the original trial, the court excluded testimony from the nurse anesthetist and the surgeon who operated about what, if any, direction the MD gave her about the type of anesthetic to use with a patient who had hepatitis in the past. The trial court allowed expert testimony on technical questions and excluded the testimony of facts in dispute. Therefore, the appellate court decided that issues of fact about what was communicated between the nurse anesthetist and the physician remained, and granted the husband's request for a new trial (*Carlsen v. Javurek*, 1975).

Inadequate informed consent can also lead to a case of negligence against an APN. In a 1976 wrongful death case, a patient died on the operating table following anesthesia given by the nurse anesthetist. The plaintiff argued that the informed consent given the patient prior to the surgery was inadequate. A Texas appeals court decided that the informed consent the patient was given did not lead to the patient's death. The plaintiff had to present evidence that the informed consent lacked critical information that would have influenced him to reject the surgery. However, the jury did not find that the plaintiff would have rejected the anesthesia if more details about the risks had been provided (*Forney v. Memorial Hospital*, 1976).

In a 1978 case, a nurse anesthetist and a first-year resident inserted an endotracheal tube into the patient's esophagus, rather than the trachea, prior to surgery for a Caesarean section. As a result, the 18-year-old patient died a few days after the Caesarean section. The nurse anesthetist was named as a codefendant with the first-year resident in anesthesiology, along with other staff at Charity Hospital in New Orleans, LA, and the jury found for the defendants. However, on appeal, the court decided that the negligence case against the nurse anesthetist and the first-year resident should be re-heard by the trial court, because evidence that negligent insertion of the tube had occurred was compelling (*Aubert v. Charity Hospital*, 1978).

In a 1979 case, a nurse anesthetist and others were sued for malpractice after an 11-year-old boy died following cardiac arrest during a cosmetic surgery for pectus excavatum, commonly known as sunken chest. The trial court found for the defendants, and this decision was affirmed on appeal, in which the only issue was whether the doctrine of *res ipsa loquitur* should have been applied by the jury. This doctrine stands for "the thing speaks for itself," in which three tests must be met: "1) the accident or injury normally does not occur in the absence of negligence; 2) there exists an absence of direct evidence to explain the activities leading to the injury; and 3) the accident or injury was caused by an agency or instrumentality within the actual or constructive control of the defendant" (*Ewen v. Baton Rouge General Hospital*, 1979, p. 174). Even though the cardiac arrest occurred during surgery, this condition can happen with or without surgical involvement and minus negligence of professionals. Therefore, the appellate court supported the trial court's judgment for the defendants.

The following year, the same defendant nurse anesthetist was named in a malpractice suit for negligent administration of Valium prior to surgery. The patient suffered phlebitis and thrombosis in the arm in which the Valium was injected. Evidence indicated that the nurse anesthetist followed the manufacturer's recommendations and the standard practice of nurse anesthetists, so the plaintiff's case failed. Interestingly, in Louisiana, the locality rule applies to generalists, not specialists, whose actions are measured in relation to other "specialists in similar circumstances" (*Mohr v. Jenkins*, 1980, p. 246). The locality rule is the idea that the standard of care is measured according to the standard in the locality in which the nurse practices, rather than a national standard. So an expert witness must be familiar with the standard in a given community, not the national standard of care, even though education of health professionals uses national standards based upon evidence-based practice (Lewis, Gohagan, & Merenstein, 2007). This creates uncertainty for health professionals about what is expected of them and may promote substandard practice (Lewis et al., 2007).

Until 1975 in Michigan, nurses could not be sued for malpractice, but the state legislature changed the law in recognition of professional judgments nurses made independently. In a 1981 case against a CRNA, the plaintiff argued that the CRNA could not be sued because a nurse had administered the anesthesia. The court did not support this argument, saying that nurse anesthetists have specialized education and certification to administer anesthesia (*Whitney v. Day*, 1981). As a side point, the standard of care to be used in Michigan was the locality rule, "in the same community" (p. 712).

In a Pennsylvania case, a nurse anesthetist and the surgeon were found jointly liable for faulty arm positioning during a gynecological procedure that resulted in supracapular nerve palsy. As was true in a previous case, the *res ipsa loquitur* analysis was applied here by the court, and in this situation, the defendants had exclusive control of the positioning of the patient, and therefore were liable for the resulting injury (*Jones v. Harrisburg Polyclinic Hospital*, 1981).

In a 1981 decision by a Louisiana court, a CRNA was found liable for improper ventilation of a patient who subsequently died. Although a physician had ordered the nurse anesthetist to insert the nasal catheter, the court found that the MD did not actually "supervise or control" the actions of the nurse anesthetist, and thus was not vicariously liable (*Hughes v. St. Paul Fire & Marine*, 1981, p. 450). The nurse anesthetist was not an employee of the physician, and argued that he was an independent contractor, which made the link between the MD and the CRNA even more tenuous.

Even when a strong case for malpractice exists, the case will be dismissed if the statute of limitations has been exceeded. A nurse anesthetist in North Dakota was named as a defendant in a suit brought by the family of a man who died from cerebral anoxia following an unsuccessful effort to administer anesthesia prior to surgery. The patient died on August 18, 1977, and the family was informed on December 9, 1977, that they had the right to sue for possible malpractice. In November of 1979, the family began the process by asking for a medical review panel to review the case, and when the judge refused to convene the panel for legal reasons, the patient's wife filed suit on December 14, 1979. In North Dakota, a suit for wrongful death must be brought 2 years from the time when the legal problem arises, in this case, the death of the patient on August 18, 1977. The statute of limitations ran for 2 years, so a suit could not be brought after August 18, 1979 (*Ness v. St. Aloisius Hospital*, 1981).

In a 1982 case, a nurse anesthetist and a physician were sued for malpractice following surgery that preceded the patient's cardiac arrest, brain damage, and subsequent death. The nurse anesthetist introduced testimony of two expert witnesses, who concluded there was no negligence. The plaintiff, however, presented an opposite opinion from an expert witness from a nearby state. The plaintiff's expert identified the following failures: "failed to make a complete preoperative evaluation of the patient before administering anesthesia…failed to adequately monitor Slayton (the patient) prior to transferring her to the recovery room…took improper steps to reverse the effects of the respiratory and cardiac arrest…failed to properly record the dosage of medication on the anesthesia record" (*Slayton v. Brunner*, 1982, p. 146). The lower court found for the defendants and dismissed the case. However, on appeal, the court reversed the judgment of the lower court by saying that the plaintiff's expert could testify on the standard of care, despite being from Oklahoma, not Arkansas. Arkansas' locality rule allowed testimony from experts who are familiar with the local standard by having accepted referrals from a similar community, consulted with health professionals from similar communities, and having health professionals with similar qualifications at their facilities. Thus, the appellate court decided there were facts in dispute that should be decided by a jury.

In a 1984 North Carolina case against a nurse anesthetist, a surgeon, assistant surgeon, and a hospital, suit was brought by a patient and her husband for malpractice, alleging that ulnar nerve damage the patient suffered following a vaginal hysterectomy was caused by poor positioning during surgery. The lower court dismissed the case, as requested by the defendants, but on appeal, the court held that issues of fact remained about the nurse anesthetist's liability for poor positioning and whether she was an employee of the hospital. Thus, the plaintiff's *res ipsa loquitur* argument was accepted (*Parks v. H. B. Perry*, 1984).

In a 1984 New York case, the husband of a patient who happened to be a registered nurse (RN) and who died from breast cancer, alleged that a physician and NP had failed to diagnose the condition in a timely manner, which led to his wife's death at age 36. The NP had seen the patient for a routine physical exam, had reviewed the records of a physician from a prior visit, and concluded that the diagnosis was fibrocystic breast disease. No evidence of the NP's negligence was provided, so the case proceeded only against the MD. The physician was held to be negligent, and the patient was awarded $950,000. The demeanor of the MD at trial did not support his argument. The court stated that because of his demeanor, the patient's testimony taken before trial was more convincing than the MD's statement of the facts (*Beckcom v. U.S.*, 1984).The demeanor was not described in any detail in the judge's opinion. However, this comment from the judge is a reminder to APNs who present evidence in court that they should be well prepared by an attorney, so that the testimony about the facts is credible.

In North Carolina, a child's mother received prenatal care from a family nurse practitioner (FNP) under the supervision of a physician. The plaintiffs, who were the child who was born with Down syndrome, the parents, and siblings, alleged that the FNP failed to inform the parents of the option of amniocentesis and genetic counseling. Had she done so, the parents would have been able to terminate the pregnancy. A case of wrongful life/wrongful birth of a child with Down syndrome was brought by the family. Ms. Dowdy was codefendant with the health care agency where she worked and with an MD in the clinic. The Supreme Court of North Carolina decided that neither claim was a viable legal claim in North Carolina. The court stated, "Whether it is better never to have been born at all than to have been born with even gross deficiencies is a mystery more properly to be left to the philosophers and the theologians. Surely, the law can assert no competence to resolve the issue, particularly in view of the very nearly uniform high value which the law and mankind has (sic) placed on human life, rather than its absence" (*Azzolino v. Dingfelder*, 1985, p. 109).

In a 1985 New York case, a patient in surgery for a gangrenous foot suffered an anoxic brain injury and subsequently died following surgery. The death certificate stated that, "the immediate cause of death was acute renal failure, due to or a consequence of broncho-pneumonia and sepsis, which was in turn due to, or a consequence of post-hypoxic encephalopathy and spastic quadraparesis" (*Rosenberg v. New York University Hospital*, 1985, p. 91). This case was brought against a nurse anesthetist, a hospital, an anesthesiologist, and a surgeon, and demonstrated the importance of a death certificate as evidence of a causal link between the negligent act and the injury (wrongful death). Thus, the death certificate can provide critical information in malpractice cases, even regarding the requirement of proximate cause (the direct and immediate cause of death).

A 1985 Washington case involved a nurse anesthetist who provided the induction prior to exploratory surgery. During the induction, the patient's airway became blocked and the nurse anesthetist was unsuccessful in clearing it. She called for help and physicians were able to open the airway, but the patient's heart stopped, and mental and physical impairments resulted. The nurse anesthetist and an anesthesiologist were sued for negligence and failure to obtain informed consent. The judge dismissed the informed consent claim, the jury found for the defendants on the negligence claim, and the plaintiff appealed. On appeal, the court said that the informed consent claim should have been allowed, because there was evidence that defendants did not provide adequate information about risks and alternatives. The *res ipsa loquitur* claim was barred in trial, but on appeal, the court said that *res ipsa loquitur* could be used in the new trial. Interestingly, the court mentioned a potentially coercive comment made by someone in the admissions process, "the little girl told me if I didn't sign it I wouldn't get the job done, so I signed the paper" (*Brown v. Dahl*, 1985, p. 786). However, the court did not rest its decision on this required element of voluntariness for informed consent.

In a 1985 California case, the actions of an NP who worked for the defendant's medical practice were evaluated by the jury according to the standard of care for physicians, as directed by the trial judge. On appeal of the verdict for the plaintiff, the Supreme Court of California said that this was an error, but not one requiring reversal of the judgment, because the judgment about negligence in this case would not have been changed (*Fein v. Permanente Medical Group*, 1985). Much evidence existed to demonstrate negligence beyond that involving the NP.

In a 1987 Louisiana case, an 11-year-old child died of aspiration pneumonia and sepsis following an episode of vomiting during the administration of anesthesia by a CRNA. Plaintiffs appealed a judgment that they as parents of a child who died in surgery for appendicitis contributed to the negligence, and that their award of damages should not be reduced by 75%. The court dropped the contributory negligence allegation by the defendants because no evidence to support this proposition was offered, and upheld the award of damages to the plaintiff (*Pierre v. Lallie Kemp Charity Hospital*, 1987). Contributory negligence refers to actions on the part of the plaintiff that partially cause the injury.

In a similar case in Nebraska in 1989 against two CRNAs, an RN was the patient who died following a hemorrhoidectomy. The CRNAs argued that because the patient was an RN, she should have known that her thyroid condition could jeopardize the use of certain anesthetics, and she didn't disclose this information during the preanesthesia assessment. The trial court had erroneously given a jury instruction about considering contributory negligence when there was no evidence presented indicating this. On appeal, the court reversed the judgment in the defendant CRNA's favor so that a new trial would omit the contributory negligence claim (*Gehre v. Coleman*, 1989). However, the court said that "there was no evidence that decedent, as a registered nurse educated in the 1920s or 1930s and retired from active nursing for more than 20 years, knew or should have known that a thyroid condition would make the administration of a particular anesthesia dangerous" (p. 38). Thus, a new trial was ordered.

Intentional Acts

Injuries to patients can come from intended actions by the APN as well as accidental actions. These cases from the 1980s involve intentional claims against APNs.

In 1984, a Massachusetts Board of Registration in Nursing suspended an RN's license, saying that she practiced midwifery without the Board's authorization, which it considered gross misconduct. The RN was not certified or formally educated as a nurse midwife, nor had the Board approved her practice as a nurse midwife. The nurse appealed the suspension, arguing that she was not practicing as a nurse midwife, but rather was practicing as a lay midwife attending home births. The Board argued that practicing lay midwifery was the unauthorized practice of medicine. Although the court agreed with the Board about the nursing licensure violation, it remanded (sent the case back) to the

Board for reconsideration of its reasons for the suspension, because the Board's ruling against the nurse was not clearly based solely upon her nursing license violation, and in Massachusetts, lay persons could practice lay midwifery (*Leigh v. Board of Registration in Nursing*, 1985).

In 1989, the Supreme Court of New York upheld the ruling of the State Commissioner of Health that a nurse anesthetist had obtained and disposed of morphine sulfate improperly and without a doctor's order. The nurse anesthetist was assessed a $7,000 fine as a civil penalty for these violations (*Damm v. Axelrod*, 1989).

Expertise and Courtroom Testimony

Courts hear testimony from parties to a lawsuit on the qualifications of expert witnesses, and allow or exclude their testimony. APNs serve as expert witnesses, but at other times, they testify about the facts of a situation that they witnessed directly. This set of cases presents situations in which the testimony of APNs was important to the resolution of the case.

In a key informed-consent case in Minnesota, *Cornfeldt v. Tongen* (1977), the Supreme Court of Minnesota decided that testimony of a nurse anesthetist should not have been excluded by the trial court. The defendants in this wrongful death case were physicians, and the issue was the adequacy of the administration of anesthesia and information the physicians had given to the patient prior to surgery. The trial court justified its exclusion of the nurse anesthetist's testimony by the fact that he was not a physician, and thus, could not testify about medical standards. However, the appellate court said that his education and licensure as a physician were not determinative, but rather if the nurse anesthetist, "otherwise had sufficient scientific and practical experience about the matter to which he would have testified, he would have been a competent expert witness" (p. 697). Interestingly, however, the court said that the exclusion of this testimony was not prejudicial to the case, and thus, its exclusion was not enough to reverse the lower court's decision by itself.

In a 1987 case in Louisiana, the plaintiff in a wrongful-death suit argued that the fact that a nurse anesthetist provided the anesthesia rather than another provider was evidence of negligence by itself. In this way, the plaintiff questioned the expertise of the nurse anesthetist. The court rejected this allegation, saying there was no link between the actions of the nurse anesthetist and the cause of the patient's death. In addition, the Joint Commission on Accreditation of Hospitals (JCAH) accreditation standards included use of nurse anesthetists in hospitals (*Garrett v. United States*, 1987).

Courts and other legal tribunals have various ways they recognize the expertise of APNs. In the settlement of an Agent Orange case in 1988, a psychiatric clinical nurse specialist (CNS) was appointed by the court to a Class Assistance Advisory Board to make recommendations about how funds from a settlement should be distributed (*In re "Agent Orange" Product Liability Litigation*, 1988). She was an Army nurse during the Vietnam War, and counseled veterans suffering from posttraumatic stress disorder (PTSD).

Similarly, in 1989, a plaintiff in New York sought to amend a case against a hospital, a surgeon, other hospital employees, and an anesthesiology practice by adding a claim for failure to inform the patient that a nurse anesthetist or medical resident might administer the anesthesia. The court denied this request, saying that informed consent need not go so far as to reveal the qualifications of personnel caring for the patient (*Abram v. Children's Hospital of Buffalo*, 1989).

In Georgia, in 1989, the testimony of an NP in a criminal case about vaginal tears during a rape was allowed by the court. The NP's education provided her with expertise on vaginal tearing. By contrast, the NP's testimony identifying the father of the 4- or 5-year-old child as the perpetrator was in error due to its status as an out-of-court statement, but due to the fact that other similar testimony was given as to the father's role in the rape, the error was ruled harmless (*Hyde v. State*, 1989).

In 1988, the Oregon Supreme Court said that the lower court had misconstrued the phrase "doctor or physician" too narrowly in claims for health care reimbursement. Instead of being limited to physicians, the phrase was inclusive of NPs (*Cook v. Worker's Compensation Department*, 1988). The Worker's Compensation statute in Oregon defined "doctor or physician" as one who is licensed to practice "one or more of the healing arts" (ORS 656.005 (12)).

Hospital and Prescriptive Privileges

Access to the services of APNs is critical to the success of their professional relationships and businesses, and therefore, admitting and prescriptive privileges are important to their status as independent providers. The following cases provide examples of judicial treatment of these evolving APN authorities and responsibilities.

In 1983, a federal District Court in California decided that a clinic that provided abortion services had grounds to sue the local medical society, a hospital, and insurance company for actions that interfered with offering the abortion services. The clinic alleged, among other things, that the defendants threatened to remove hospital privileges of clinic MDs and NPs. The court reviewed various legal grounds that could be alleged, and concluded that a case could be made for interference by the defendants with the right of privacy of clinic clients (*Chico Feminist Women's Health Center v. Butte Glenn Medical Society*, 1983).

In 1989, a federal District Court in Georgia dismissed a case brought by a Certified Nurse Midwife (CNM) against a hospital. The CNM alleged that the hospital violated the Sherman Anti-Trust Act and the First Amendment by not allowing her access to patients in the hospital and for expressing her views about natural birth. She had established a nurse-midwifery business, and doctors at the hospital stated publicly that she lacked adequate back-up from physicians and otherwise provided inadequate care, including her statements in support of home birth. The hospital refused to allow her staff privileges. She then sued the hospital for restraint of trade under the antitrust act, violation of her free speech, and intentional infliction of emotional distress. The court decided the dispute was a private one between the CNM and the physicians, and therefore, the hospital was justified in doing what it did to preserve the safety of its clients. Her claims did not rise to the level of harm to the public nor were the actions of the physicians egregious or harassing. In addition, the antitrust action was dismissed because the hospital exercised its right of immunity as a public hospital (*Sweeney v. Athens Regional Medical Center*, Feb. 1989).

In a subsequent case by the CNM in the same court involving the same parties, but focused on the two women's health clinics and the physicians, the decision was different. The court found that the CNM did present evidence of an impact on interstate commerce, a conspiracy to restrain her teaching and home-birth practice, and an injury to her practice as a result of illegal actions by the clinics and MDs, and facts supportive of intentional infliction of emotional distress and slander. Thus, the defendants' motion to dismiss the case was not supported (*Sweeney v. Athens Regional Medical Center*, March 1989).

Also in 1989, a federal court in West Virginia threw out an antitrust case brought by an NP and an MD against a hospital for denying them hospital privileges. The court pointed out that an impact on interstate commerce required in an antitrust claim was not alleged in the plaintiff's case (*Tempkin v. Lewis-Gale Hospital, Inc.*, 1989).

By 1989, 26 jurisdictions granted prescriptive authority to nurses in two categories: states in which nurses could prescribe independently of physicians, and those in which nurses were obligated to collaborate with physicians to prescribe (Hadley, 1989). North Carolina led the way, with licensure of nurses instituted in 1903, prescriptive authority granted in 1975, and in organizing the first educational programs for NPs in the late 1960s and early 1970s at the University of North Carolina at Chapel Hill (Hadley, 1989). However, NPs in North Carolina to this day are restricted by the requirements that both medical and nursing boards must approve them to practice, and a collaborative relationship with one specific physician is required.

In summary, roles and privileges of APNs expanded in scope from the 1950s through the 1980s. APNs were more frequently discussed by name in court opinions over time, with the standards expected of them more clearly defined in the areas of assessment, diagnosis, and interventions. They were more often considered expert witnesses in the areas of their practice, and APNs also began to bring antitrust lawsuits to defend their business interests.

RELATIONSHIPS BETWEEN APNs AND PHYSICIANS

Just as standards of care have increasingly recognized the authority and the corresponding legal and ethical responsibilities of APNs to their patients, the relationships between APNs and physicians have evolved toward increasing independence but continuing collaboration between the two disciplines. The following cases demonstrate these APN/MD relationship changes during the 1970s and 1980s.

Antitrust

Businesses are encouraged to compete with one another in truthful, reasonable ways, but restraint of trade, monopolization, and other anti-competitive efforts are against the law. Legal actions taken against businesses that fix prices with other businesses or take other actions that keep others from competing fall into the antitrust area of the law. Health care businesses are no exception to this rule, in part because of the large portion of our economy that is involved in these businesses (Jacobs, 1986). In a 1987 case in Mississippi, a CRNA sued a hospital for interfering with her business as an independent contractor for anesthesia services. She was given 60% of the payments the hospital received for her services, whereas a dentist who provided anesthesia for the hospital received 100% of the reimbursement. The federal court said a case against the hospital could proceed as an antitrust case (*Wicker v. Union County General Hospital*, 1987).

In *Nurse Midwifery Associates v. Hibbett*, a 1990 case in Tennessee, a nurse midwifery practice and a physician who provided supervision and other services for the practice sued physicians, hospitals, and an insurance company owned and run by physicians for conspiracy in restraint of trade. In addition to denying the nurse midwives staff privileges at the hospitals, the insurance company refused to renew the supervising physician a continuation of his malpractice policy. Because the nurse midwives could not obtain other physician supervision, they closed their practice and brought this suit. The lower court found for the defendants on most of the claims, but on appeal, the court remanded the case for presentation of evidence on the claim of conspiracy between the physicians and the insurance company to eliminate the physician's malpractice coverage. In an antitrust case, an entity or party cannot conspire with itself, so if the physicians were agents of the hospital, they could not conspire with the hospital. But they could conspire with each other and the insurance company, because they were in competition with each other and the insurance company was not their employer. One interesting quote from the testimony demonstrates the negative attitudes one of the physicians had toward nurse midwives: "If nurse midwives started delivering babies, the next thing they would want to do is heart surgery" (p. 609).

Noncompete Clauses

Health care practices, like other businesses, protect their interests by expecting new employees to sign noncompete covenants. These contracts bind the employee who leaves employment not to work for a period of time within a certain radius of the employer's business location. As courts construe these agreements narrowly, and sometimes change their terms if considered unreasonable, the terms should be explicit and time-limited. Because some states do not allow noncompete clauses, APNs need to consult with attorneys as they enter into employment contracts (The American Association of Nurse Attorneys, 2005).

A CNM was employed by an Illinois practice in 1981, and terminated her employment in 1985. In a lawsuit against her by the practice, a practice official testified that an oral noncompete covenant had been accepted by the CNM when she entered employment. However, the CNM said no such oral covenant had been offered to or accepted by her. The plaintiff asked the court to issue preliminary injunctions against the CNM to keep her from conducting her new practice within the 10-mile radius of the practice, not to use trade secrets (patients' names and other identifying information), and practice medicine without a license (unfair trade practices). The lower court denied this request, so the plaintiff appealed. The Illinois appellate court agreed with the lower court on the first and third issues, but said the preliminary injunction should be issued for the trade secrets claim, because the CNM herself testified that she had copied names and information about the patients to contact them (*Prentice Medical Corporation v. Todd*, 1986).

Evidence wasn't strong enough in the case for the noncompete agreement to be supported, but if it had been in writing, the court may have supported the plaintiffs. Noncompete covenants also can be used by APNs who own their own businesses, and where the structure and use of these covenants are important to sound business practice.

Insurance/Third-Party Payment

Poor reimbursement rates for APN services from public or private sources, such as insurance companies, were challenged by APNs from the beginning. As a result of these concerns, APNs advocated for studies that compared effectiveness of their services with that of MDs. The earliest major study by the U.S. Office of Technology Assessment in 1986 demonstrated the strength and comparability of the APN primary care service (Office of Technology Assessment, 1986).

When an APN buys his or her own professional liability policy, the insurance company may raise questions that slow resolution of the case. In a 1973 wrongful death case in New York, two insurance companies, one defending the hospitals and the other defending the CRNA, asked the court for a declaratory judgment about which policy should pay for the damages as primary insurer. The CRNA's malpractice company alleged that the CRNA had acted beyond her scope of practice, practicing medicine without a license. Because this issue was raised, the New York court sent the case back to the trial court to resolve the original malpractice case (*Argonaut Insurance Company v. Continental Insurance Company*, 1978).

In a malpractice case against a nurse anesthetist, her insurance company and that of the hospital sought a declaratory judgment from the court about which company might be responsible financially for the nurse anesthetist's actions. Her insurance policy was paid for by the anesthesiologist, and the hospital said it would not cover her as she was not an employee of the hospital. A New York court sent the case back to the lower court to find facts about whether the contract had been transferred from one anesthesiologist to another, and the effectiveness of the cancellation notice to the nurse anesthetist (*Benedictine Hospital v. Hospital Underwriters Mutual Insurance Company*, 1984). This case demonstrates the risks associated with not owning one's own malpractice policy.

In the mid-1980s, the insurance company providing blanket professional liability insurance for nurse midwives went bankrupt. The American College of Nurse Midwives advocated for another insurance company, but couldn't find a company to provide the coverage. However, shortly thereafter in 1986, several insurance companies joined together in a consortium to provide the coverage (Lefkin, 1988).

Supervision by Physicians

Supervision of a nurse anesthetist was at issue in a North Carolina negligence case. The nurse anesthetist anesthetized the patient prior to surgery for laminectomy. A few minutes into surgery, the patient's blood pressure and pulse dropped to zero, and the anesthesiologist was called and came within a minute to resuscitate the patient. However, the patient had suffered brain damage and died a few days later. Under North Carolina law, nurse anesthetists could only administer anesthesia under direct supervision and direction by the physician. As a result, the defendants lost their motion for *summary judgment* (a legal decision that the facts do not justify further arguments in the case) (*Bentley v. Langley*, 1978).

In another 1978 case with a different result, a Louisiana court concluded that a nurse anesthetist did not have to be under the direct control of a physician. She selected and properly administered the anesthetics. The patient died after an adverse reaction to Anectine and subsequent cardiac arrest. The defendant hospital and physicians won this case, as no improper procedures or poor judgments were used (*Brown v. Allen Sanitarium*, 1978).

In a 1982 Ohio malpractice case, the court decided a surgeon had the right of control over the nurse anesthetist who was not employed by the surgeon. Also, the surgeon stated that he had instructed the nurse anesthetist about the procedures to follow. Therefore, he could be held liable for her actions (*Baird v. Sickler*, 1982).

In a Missouri case in 1983, several NPs and MDs sought a declaratory injunction from the court to clarify whether the actions of the NPs were practicing medicine without a license. A declaratory judgment is a decision by a court that determines the rights and relationships between the parties without ordering specific actions or outcomes, such as penalties. NPs were following standing orders and protocols written by the doctors, and the orders varied by each NP, which indicated unique approaches to the skills and abilities of each NP. The court noted the new definition of professional nursing in state law and changes in the field of advanced practice nursing, and decided that the actions of the NPs fell clearly within nursing practice, and thus, did not constitute the practice of medicine. Numerous friend of the court briefs (amicus briefs) were submitted in favor of or opposed to the position of the plaintiff NPs and MDs (*Sermchief v. Gonzales*, 1983). Clearly, the case was a breakthrough for nursing autonomy in terms of allowing independent judgment.

Sometimes, a medical licensure board attempts to regulate nursing practice too tightly, as happened in Arkansas in 1984. In this case, the medical board imposed a requirement on physicians who employed or collaborated with NPs that they could hire or collaborate with no more than two NPs at the same time. Working with more than two NPs would be considered malpractice. The state nurses association sought a declaratory judgment from the court that this regulation was invalid. The lower court upheld the regulation, but on appeal, the Supreme Court of Arkansas reversed the decision of the lower court, striking down the regulation as inconsistent with similar regulation of physicians who worked with physicians' assistants (PAs) as interfering with the need for NPs in the state, and because the medical board could not create a nonstatutory restriction on a physician's license. A basic premise of American law, the separation of powers between the executive branch, in this case the licensing board, and the legislative branch, had been violated (*Arkansas State Nurses Association v. Arkansas State Medical Board*, 1984).

In a 1985 Georgia case, a student nurse anesthetist, a PA who supervised her during the administration of anesthesia, several anesthesiologists, and others were sued by the family of a woman who suffered cardiac arrest and brain damage following surgery for tubal ligation. The student nurse anesthetist used a mask rather than an endotracheal tube, which an expert testified was not standard procedure. A Georgia statute specified that a CRNA could administer anesthesia only under the "direction and responsibility" of an anesthesiologist [O.C.G.A. § 43-26-9(6)(b)]. Because a student nurse anesthetist had administered the anesthesia under no supervision by an anesthesiologist, the Georgia statute was violated on its face. The type of violation is known as *negligence per se*, and results in a shift of the burden of proof to the defendants. The lower court supported the *negligence per se* ruling, and on appeal, the Georgia Supreme Court agreed (*Central Anesthesia Associates v. Worthy, Castro v. Worthy, Moorehead v. Worthy, Executive Committee of the Baptist Convention v. Worthy*, 1985).

Courts of law are not the only legal forums facing questions about supervisory relationships between APNs and physicians. In a 1986 Louisiana case brought by the medical licensure board against the nursing licensure board, the medical board prevailed on a statute of limitations question. The nursing board planned to eliminate the phrase, "under the direction of a physician," from its rules for NPs. The medical board objected and sued the nursing board. The nursing board argued that the medical board should have brought suit within 30 days of the change in the rule. The trial court agreed, and the medical board appealed. On appeal, the court reversed the trial court's ruling because no 30-day limit was specified in the statute (*Louisiana State Medical Society v. Louisiana State Board of Nursing*, 1986).

In a 1986 wrongful death case against a VA hospital, including a nurse anesthetist employee of the VA and an anesthesiologist who worked for a private anesthesiology practice, the court held that the VA could be found liable for the acts of its agent, the nurse anesthetist, and the anesthesiologist. Just because the anesthesiologist was an employee of the outside practice, the VA could not shield itself from liability for his actions. The VA hospital held itself out to the public as a full-service hospital, and thus induced the public to rely on the VA's responsibility for acts of the anesthesiologist (*Gamble v. United States v. University Anesthesiologists*, 1986). So, if CRNAs are part of a private practice, hospitals that they work in may still be responsible for their actions.

In a 1987 Florida case, a CRNA was found by the court *not* to be under supervision or control of the obstetrician who was performing a cesarean. Thus, the surgeon was not responsible for the improper insertion of the endotracheal tube, the aspiration of vomitus, brain damage, and subsequent death of the mother. Although the surgeon had the choice of anesthesia, he did not control the procedures used by the CRNA (*Fortson v. McNamara*, 1987).

As time moves forward, courts allow more responsibility to rest with CRNAs and less to those physicians or other entities involved in surgery. An employment agency that assigned the CRNA to work at a hospital was not supervising or controlling her work in the hospital, so was not held liable for her administration of anesthesia (*Joyce v. National Medical Registry, Inc.,* 1988). And the same year, a CRNA and student nurse anesthetist were named as defendants in a malpractice case, in which the student and the CRNA who supervised her placed an endotracheal tube in the esophagus, and the patient was deprived of oxygen for 12 minutes and was brain-damaged. The case was dismissed by the lower court, but on appeal, the Tennessee court of appeals held that the physicians in the operating room and the anesthesiologist, who was not on duty, would not be liable for the actions of the nurse anesthetists (*Parker v. Vanderbilt,* 1988). Growing independence has its downsides.

And in another case yielding increasingly independent responsibility for a mistake in administration of anesthesia by a nurse anesthetist, and not the anesthesia corporation that employed her, a Florida court refused to grant attorneys fees to the corporation that had employed her, commenting that none of the physician shareholders in the corporation had directly supervised the nurse anesthetist, and therefore were not liable for her acts (*Gershuny v. Martin McFall Messenger Anesthesia Professional Association,* 1989).

In summary, prior to 1990, the relationships between APNs and physicians moved away from the supervisory, and toward increasing collaboration. APNs began to join with physicians in lawsuits to resolve antitrust claims. APNs also learned about problems with insurance companies where company actions at times slowed resolution of APN claims for coverage. Likewise, noncompete clauses became a source of concern for APNs who left a practice that required the noncompete agreement. During this period of time, cases demonstrated increasing independence of APNs from physician oversight, and a corresponding increase in sole responsibility for APN actions.

SUMMARY

The practice of APNs between 1950 and 1990 changed from limited autonomy to increasing levels of responsibility for interventions and patient care results. "In the late 70's and 80's the increasingly competitive health care market in conjunction with the professional/autonomy concerns of NPs account for APNs' seeking autonomous practice, unfettered economic reimbursement, hospital privileges, and prescriptive authority" (Inglis & Kjervik, 1993, p. 196). Most published negligence cases during this time involved errors made by nurse anesthetists in the administration of anesthetics, positioning of patients during the administration, and information shared with the team or the patient. Successful defenses to malpractice cases were arguments that violations of statute of limitations had occurred, customary practice standards were met, no legal grounds for the case existed (wrongful life/birth), and no causal connection existed between intervention and injury. Intentional acts of an APN were found in cases in which questions of misrepresentation of one's professional credentials and improper use of controlled substances existed.

Other cases involving professional status, such as interpretation of third-party reimbursement statutes as inclusive of APNs and the expertise of an APN to testify in civil and criminal cases, were found. Cases addressing APNs' hospital and prescriptive privileges pointed to the importance of the patient's right of privacy, the APNs claims of antitrust violations, slander, and intentional infliction of emotional distress.

Cases questioning the control or supervision of APNs by physicians continued in importance during this time. Claims of conspiracy in constraint of trade were accepted by courts, as were suits to clarify which insurance carrier would be responsible to pay damages for the APN and the validity of noncompete covenants required by medical practices. The general trend was toward increasing responsibility of APNs for their professional actions without concurrent liability of the physician or physician practices. This trend has continued to the present day with, for instance, all states now allowing prescriptive authority to NPs, Georgia having been the last state to allow NPs to prescribe (Ritter & Hansen-Turton, 2008).

Yet the attitudes of physician organizations about APN practice, although somewhat improved, continue to reflect their equivocal view of APN practice. For instance, a 2009 policy statement of the American College of Physicians entitled, "Nurse Practitioners in Primary Care," states the physician should be head of the health care team, that NP skills are not equivalent to the MD's, that studies showing comparable quality of care between NPs and MDs should be viewed with caution, that patients need "access to a personal physician who accepts responsibility for their entire health, working in collaboration with non-physician clinicians involved in caring for the patient" (American College of Physicians, 2009, p. 13), and that NPs should not replace primary care medical practice. In light of the fact that according to the Pearson report (Pearson, 2009), 13 states have no restrictions on NPs' diagnosis, treatment, and prescriptions; and 10 other states have no restrictions on diagnosis and treatment; the effort to obtain greater autonomy for

APNs is gaining momentum, and physicians' efforts to require supervision and collaboration are eroding. Studies continue to show cost-effectiveness, patient satisfaction with the care of APNs, and in some ways, more satisfaction with care (Horrocks, Anderson, & Salisbury, 2002; Karlowitz & McMurray, 2000; Mullinex & Bucholtz, 2009; Needleman & Minnick, 2009).

KEY POINTS

1. From the 1950s through the 1980s, advanced practice nursing changed from limited autonomy to increasing levels of responsibility, and the law reflected this trend.
2. Physician attitudes toward advanced practice nursing gradually improved during this time, but continue to display equivocation.
3. By 2009, according to the Pearson report, 13 states had no restrictions on NPs' diagnosis, treatment, and prescriptions, and 10 states had no restrictions on diagnosis and treatment, demonstrating increased legal autonomy.
4. Studies continue to show cost-effectiveness and patient satisfaction with APN practice.

REFERENCES

American College of Physicians. (2009). *Nurse practitioners in primary care* (Policy monograph). Philadelphia: Author.

Baer, E. D. (1993). Philosophical and historical bases of primary care nursing. In M. D. Mezey & D. O. McGivern (Eds.), *Nurses, nurse practitioners: Evolution to advanced practice*. New York: Springer Publishing Company.

Bartter, K. (2001). *Ethical issues in advanced nursing practice*. Boston: Butterworth-Heinemann.

Hadley, E. (1989). Nurses and prescriptive authority: A legal and economic analysis. *American Journal of Law & Medicine, 15,* 245–300.

Horrocks, S., Anderson, E., & Salisbury, C. (2002). Systematic review of whether nurse practitioners working in primary care can provide equivalent care to doctors. *British Medical Journal, 324*(7341), 819–823.

Inglis, A., & Kjervik, D. (1993). Empowerment of advanced practice nurses: Regulation reform needed to increase access to care. *Journal of Law, Medicine & Ethics, 21*(2), 193–205.

Jacobs, W. (1986). Examining collusive conduct in health care markets: A law enforcement prospective, *Federal Bar News & Journal, 33,* 334.

Karlowitz, M. G., & McMurray, J. L. (2000). Comparison of neonatal nurse practitioners and pediatric residents' care of extremely low-birth-weight infants. *Archives of Pediatrics & Adolescent Medicine, 154*(11), 1123–1126.

Lefkin, P. (1988). Shattering some myths on the insurance liability crisis: A comment on the article by Clarke, Warren-Boulton, Smith, and Simon. *Yale Journal on Regulation, 5*, 417.

Lewis, M. H., Gohagan, J. K., & Merenstein, D. J. (2007). The locality rule and the physician's dilemma: Local medical practices vs. the national standard of care. *Journal of the American Medical Association, 297*(23), 2633–2637.

McGivern, D. O. (1993). The evolution to advanced nursing practice. In M. D. Mezey & D. O. McGivern (Eds.), *Nurses, nurse practitioners: Evolution to advanced practice.* New York: Springer Publishing Company.

Mullinex, C., & Bucholtz, D. (2009). Role and quality of nurse practitioner practice: A policy issue. *Nursing Outlook, 57*(2), 93–98.

Needleman, J., & Minnick, A. F. (2009). Anesthesia provider model, hospital resources, and maternal outcomes. *Health Services Research, 44*(2), 464–482.

Office of Technology Assessment. (1986). *Nurse practitioners, physician assistants, and certified nurse midwives: A policy analysis* (Health Technology Case 37). Washington, DC: Author.

Pearson, L. (2009). The Pearson report. *American Journal for Nurse Practitioners, 13*(2), 8–82.

Ritter, A., & Hansen-Turton, T. (2008). Primary care paradigm shift: An overview of the state-level legal framework governing nurse practitioner practice. *Health Lawyer, 20*(4), 21–28.

The American Association of Nurse Attorneys. (2005). *Business and legal guidebook for nurse practitioners.* Columbus, OH: Author.

TABLE OF CASES

Abram v. Children's Hospital of Buffalo, 151 A.D.2d 972, 542 N.Y.S.2d 418 (1989).

Argonaut Insurance Company v. Continental Insurance Company, 63 A.D.2d 927, 406 N.Y.S.2d 96 (1978).

Arkansas State Nurses Association v. Arkansas State Medical Board, 283 Ark. 366, 677 S.W.2d 293 (1984).

Aubert v. Charity Hospital, 363 So.2d 1223 (1978).

Azzolino v. Dingfelder, 315 N.C. 103, 109, 337 S.E.2d, 528, 533 (1985).

Baird v. Sickler, 69 Ohio St.2d 652, 433 N.E.2d 593 (1982).

Beckcom v. U.S., 584 F. Supp. 1471 (1984).

Bentley v. Langley, 39 N.C. App. 20, 249 S.E.2d 481 (1978).

Benedictine Hospital v. Hospital Underwriters Mutual Insurance Company, 103 A.D.2d 553, 481 N.Y.

Brown v. Allen Sanitarium, 364 So.2d 661 (1978).

Brown v. Dahl, 41 Wash. App. 565, 705 P.2d 781 (1985).

Carlsen v. Javurek, 526 F.2d 202 (1975).

Central Anesthesia Associates v. Worthy, Castro v. Worthy, Moorehead v. Worthy, Executive Committee of the Baptist Convention v. Worthy, 254 Ga. 728, 333 S.E.2d 829 (1985).

Chico Feminist Women's Health Center v. Butte Glenn Medical Society, 557 F. Supp. 1190 (1983).

Cook v. Worker's Compensation Department, 758 P.2d 854, 306 Or. 134 (1988).

Cornfeldt v. Tongen, 262 N.W.2d 684 (1977).

Damm v. Axelrod, 148 A.D.2d 974, 539 N.Y.S.2d 210 (1989).

Ewen v. Baton Rouge General Hospital, 378 So.2d 172 (1979).

Fein v. Permanente Medical Group, 38 Cal.3d 137, 695 P.2d 665, 211 Cal. Rptr. 368 (1985).

Forney v. Memorial Hospital, 543 S.W.2d 705 (1976).

Fortson v. McNamara, 508 So.2d 35 (1987).

Gamble v. United States v. University Anesthesiologists, 648 F. Supp. 438 (1986).

Garrett v. United States, 667 F. Supp. 1147 (1987).

Gehre v. Coleman, 233 Neb. 32, 443 N.W.2d 606 (1989).

Gore v. United States, 229 F. Supp. 547 (1964).

Gershuny v. Martin McFall Messenger Anesthesia Professional Association, 539 So.2d 1131 (1989).

Hughes v. St. Paul Fire & Marine, 401 So.2d 448 (1981).

Hyde v. State, 189 Ga. App. 727, 377 S.E.2d 187 (1989).

In re "Agent Orange" Product Liability Litigation, 689 F. Supp. 1250 (1988). S.2d 813 (1984).

Jones v. Harrisburg Polyclinic Hospital, 496 Pa. 465, 437 A.2d 1134 (1981).

Joyce v. National Medical Registry, Inc., 170 Ill. App.3d 141, 524 N.E.2d 243, 120 Ill. Dec. 478 (1988).

Kemalyan v. Henderson, 45 Wash.2d 693, 277 P.2d 372 (1954).

Leigh v. Board of Registration in Nursing, 395 Mass. 670, 481 N.E.2d 1347 (1985).

Louisiana State Medical Society v. Louisiana State Board of Nursing, 484 So.2d 903 (1986).

Mohr v. Jenkins, 393 So.2d 245 (1980).

Ness v. St. Aloisius Hospital, 301 N.W. 657 (1981).

Nurse Midwifery Associates v. Hibbett, 918 F.2d 605 (1990).

Parker v. Vanderbilt, 767 S.W.2d. 412 (1988).

Parks v. H. B. Perry, 68 N.C. App. 202, 314 S.E.2d 287 (1984).

Pierre v. Lallie Kemp Charity Hospital, 515 So.2d 614 (1987).

Prentice Medical Corporation v. Todd, 145 Ill. App.3d 692, 495 N.E.2d 1044, 99 Ill. Dec. 309 (1986).

Rosenberg v. New York University Hospital, 128 Misc.2d 90, 488 N.Y.S.2d 599 (1985).

Sermchief v. Gonzales, 660 S.W.2d 683 (1983).

Slayton v. Brunner, 276 Ark. 143, 633 S.W.2d 29 (1982).

Sweeney v. Athens Regional Medical Center, 705 F. Supp. 1556 (Feb. 1989).

Sweeney v. Athens Regional Medical Center, 709 F. Supp. 1563 (Mar. 1989).

Tempkin v. Lewis-Gale Hospital, Inc., 1989 WL 161163 (W.D.Va.) (1989).

Whitney v. Day, 100 Mich. App. 707, 300 N.W.2d 380 (1981).

Wicker v. Union County General Hospital, 673 F. Supp. 177 (1987).

Yorston v. Pennell, 397 Pa. 28, 153 A.2d 255 (1959).

2

The Interface of Nursing Law and Ethics

DIANE KJERVIK

Liberal societies ought not to be in the business of specifying individuals' conceptions of the good, but they ought to be in the business of enabling their citizens to live a good life.

—*E. Blacksher*

As science pays increasing attention to the needs of diverse and underserved populations, the intersection among race, financial status, gender, age, and other crucial characteristics becomes a vital point of attention for advanced practice nurses (APNs). Ethical issues, such as justice, power, and choice, reside at this intersection, and if fully understood, provide enlightenment about the realities of living life as a person with any of these characteristics. For instance, older persons are vulnerable because of physical limitations that restrict their access to health services and social support and, if cognitively impaired, their ability to navigate networks that are critical to self-efficacy and self-esteem. The purpose of this chapter is to review ethical frameworks related to nursing law, to explore the tensions that exist among ethical approaches, and to examine the sometimes conflicting duties of APNs to patients, nursing, professional colleagues, and professional organizations. Underpinning this analysis are the realities of the lives of patients and other populations served by APNs, including the meaning of choice for those who are vulnerable. Also, approaches that APNs may use to promote autonomous decision making by patients in the context of their connections to the community will be suggested. Preventive ethics (noticing and taking action on ethical problems before they arise) as described by Grace (2009), and the similar path to prevention of legal problems (risk management), reduce the emotional toll on those involved and other costs associated with unresolved ethical conflicts or litigation.

COMMON ETHICAL FRAMEWORKS

For persons who are vulnerable because of health status, economic strength, gender, race, or other reasons, ethical questions arise as to how power shifts affect the vulnerable person or group. For instance, APNs have a responsibility to advocate for policy change to improve the lives of persons in poverty (Grace, 2009). Persons might be in poverty over many years, suddenly as a result of catastrophic illness, or for longer periods of time as cognitive impairment develops from diseases such as Alzheimer's disease or arteriosclerosis. Social mores may also change, placing people outside their usual support systems. For instance, in the United States, care by extended families used to be common, but in recent years, the immediate family typically cares for itself without benefit of support from uncles, aunts, cousins, and often grandparents, as well. And, by way of another example, in India, where in the past older persons were cared for by their extended families, now they are more often left to fend for themselves when they are most vulnerable (Goering, 2007).

Changes in social mores such as these may result in poverty, reducing the individual's resilience to disease and exercise of his or her life choices. An overview of ethical approaches as described by Beauchamp and Childress (2009) provides the framework in which the actions of health care providers can be developed, tested, and evaluated. Morality refers to general norms about conduct that are widely shared within the community. Ethics refers to ways of examining the moral life, either in terms of what should be done (normative ethics), what is being done and believed (descriptive ethics), or how we analyze the meaning of ethical reasoning and language (metaethics) (Beauchamp & Childress, 2009).

Deontology

In the deontological view of ethics, principles such as autonomy, beneficence, and justice are applied in specific situations. One's duty in the situation is described as the categorical imperative, the idea that one should act in such a way that the action could become universal (Beauchamp & Childress, 2009). For instance, much concern for the individual's right to make health care decisions autonomously is a cornerstone of ethics in the United States, and should be evaluated in patients as they become less able for physical, psychological, or other reasons to function at their previous levels.

Consequentialism (Teleology)

In the consequentialist view of ethics, the endpoints, or *telos*, of one's actions are emphasized in deciding whether one's conduct is right or wrong. Utilitarianism is the most common theory in this perspective, focuses on well-being (the balance of positive value over negative value), and is often described as the, "greatest good for the greatest number of people" (Beauchamp & Childress, 2009). Utilitarians evaluate outcomes such as happiness, friendship, health, or personal relationships as valuable (Beauchamp & Childress, 2009). The endpoint matters more than the motives of the actor to respect autonomy or act with the good of the person in mind (beneficence). In a recent study of nurse practitioners (NPs), the investigators who interviewed both new and experienced NPs to ascertain their moral concerns and distress found that concerns about the greater good were one of five areas identified (Godfrey & Smith, 2002). Specifically, NPs focused on the individual patient in front of them, and felt frustrated that societal issues could not be dealt with by them in their practices.

Casuistry

Beauchamp and Childress (2009) refer to casuistry as "bottom-up thinking" (p. 376). This inductive approach examines each case in depth for every detail, and then identifies patterns that evolve over time and compares them with the present case. So when an APN makes a decision, the goodness or rightness of this choice is assessed in terms of what this APN and other APNs have done in these specific circumstances. When a court case develops that involves the APN, judicial law operates in this fashion by examining the specific details of the case and how these details can be distinguished from other cases. Based on precedents from previous cases, the court's judgment is used by other courts making decisions about similar cases (Beauchamp & Childress, 2009). Thus, documentation in the health care record of APN assessments made and actions taken are very important to complete, from both ethical and legal standpoints.

Communitarianism

This approach to ethics emphasizes the welfare of the group above the welfare of the individual. So, preservation of groups such as the family, professions, organizations, and society is used to analyze the goodness of someone's conduct (Beauchamp & Childress, 2009). In the United States, individualism and freedom are valued highly, and thus, autonomy of action is typically placed above the good of the group. However, in several European countries, presumed consent to obtain organs for transplant is accepted policy (Beauchamp & Childress, 2009). Presumed consent laws allow for removal of organs for transplant unless an objection is formally recorded, thus favoring the good of the community.

Ethic of Care

Building and maintaining relationships among individuals is the focus of care-based ethics. Thus, the rightness of the conduct is evaluated in terms of whether the action improves the relationships within a support network. This ethical orientation emphasizes the traits valued in personal relationships, such as, "sympathy, compassion, fidelity, and love" (Beauchamp & Childress, 2009, p. 36). The ethic of care was used by half of the NPs in one study (Rittenbach, 2005), and is viewed as a link between the science and art of nursing (Meadows, 2007). Beauchamp and Childress (2009) consider the ethic of care as falling within virtue ethics, due to its focus on the character and intentions of the health professional.

Virtue Ethics

Character traits of individuals, such as integrity, trustworthiness, compassion, discernment, and conscientiousness, are considered the five focal virtues for health professionals (Beauchamp & Childress, 2009). Passive virtues in nursing, such as obedience and submission, were valued early in the profession, and more recently, active virtues reflective of the advocacy role of nurses (respectfulness, considerateness, justice, persistence, and courage) are displayed in nursing (Beauchamp & Childress, 2009). Grace (2009) adds that in their supervisory roles, APNs are also required to show virtues of leadership and cooperation.

These approaches to ethics are not mutually exclusive. APNs should identify ethical dilemmas they face, and then consider each of these approaches using "reflective equilibrium," as described by Beauchamp and Childress (2009, p. 381), to achieve a coherent organization of their own beliefs. The goal of this process "is to match, prune, and adjust considered judgments and their specifications to render them coherent with the premises of our most general moral commitments" (p. 382). When APNs develop this coherent set of beliefs, they will be more able to merge ethical commitments into their professional judgments about patient care comfortably.

ETHICAL UNDERPINNINGS OF LEGAL ANALYSIS

As Grace (2009) points out, "from a philosophical stance, good practice is equivalent to ethical practice" (p. 57). However, the concept of the "good" or "right" behavior does not translate automatically to the ability of APNs to accomplish their goals. Ethical orientations guide actions of health professionals, but legal decisions embody policy choices made by our society, and many of these policy choices do not provide adequate support to act beneficently (promoting the good) for those who are vulnerable or uninsured, groups often served by APNs. American law emphasizes differences among people such as age, race, ethnicity, but as Minow (1990) points out, differences should not be the only concern in legal thought; relationships among people should also be considered. She says, "I advocate a shift in the paradigm we use to conceive of difference, a shift from a focus on the distinctions between people to a focus on relationships within which we notice and draw distinctions" (p. 15). Minow's suggested approach to legal decision making falls in line with the ethic of care, but incorporates individualism (autonomy), as well. As she says, "But I do not reject all that the prior frames of thought have offered; I suggest a dialectical approach connecting a renewed interest in relationships to the prior frameworks that emphasized rights and distinctions between people" (p. 15). To accomplish this goal, Minow suggests, "challenging and transforming the unstated norm used for comparisons, taking the perspective of the traditionally excluded or marginal group, disentangling equality from its attachment to a norm that has the effect of unthinking exclusion, and treating everyone as though he or she were different" (p. 16). Thus, the vital analytical approach akin to casuistry identifies the unstated norms expected of vulnerable persons, which, in the health care context, become standards by which the "normal" person is measured, and then the individual situation faced by each person is factored into the approach to be taken. This individual tailoring is understood clearly by APNs, but policy makers often overlook the distinctions as they create law affecting large populations.

Some confusion exists as to the extent of legal involvement with ethical matters, particularly with legal advocacy. Law is not limited to advocacy of individual clients in the judicial system, as Grace (2009) states. The legal system also includes legislative and executive branch actions which result in wide-reaching societal impact. Lawyers become legislators or officials in executive branch agencies such as the Department of Health and Human Services or the Food and Drug Administration, and both of these areas of law require advocacy for constituents (legislative) or policy choices mandated in statute (executive branch). If law related to health care is to be effective, it needs to use means testing and other measures of difference among individuals, and not rely on stereotypic views of groups of patients. To better inform law makers, research on variations in factors that affect health care choices and associated costs must be tailored to examine types of services and resources needed, types of disabilities, functional limitations, demand for care, and the context of care (Parker & Thorslund, 2007). In this way, ethical perspectives drawn from research findings based on the realities of vulnerable populations can be fused with legal decisions. One example of recent legislative change that attends to individual difference is that of apology for medical or nursing errors. As reported by Sack (2008), the number of lawsuits against hospitals and providers has dropped since the apologies for errors and offers of fair compensation have been made. Thus, the apology for specific actions taken by specific providers to a given patient is tailored to specific needs and circumstances, thus reducing costs of litigation. This type of law reflects care-based, compassionate, and beneficent ethical perspectives, as well as the virtues of integrity and honesty.

PROMOTING PATIENT AUTONOMY

Autonomy refers to self-chosen action, and is viewed as self-determination in the law. Autonomy may be compromised when a person is cognitively impaired or is a minor. Also, health concerns of the poor, such as physical and mental health, sometimes obscure the moral "health" of the individual. As Blacksher (2002) explains, moral agency may be impaired, resulting in less ability to make authentic decisions on one's own behalf. As she states, "the 'injuries' to the moral self refer not only to the diminished autonomy of choices and choosers, but to the source of both: one's identity or 'sense of self' " (p. 460). She suggests that each of us may have an obligation to promote the agency of others, similar to the responsible assertive behavior proposed by Lange and Jakubowski (1976). The APN is in the position not only to help patients to develop and express their choices, but to help others who interact with the patient to develop these skills, as well.

One's moral agency precedes one's ability to exercise other forms of power, such as promoting public policy that supports the needs of those who are vulnerable. For instance, Maliski, Clerkin, and Litwin (2004) have developed nursing interventions for low-income older men with prostate cancer that improve their self-efficacy. The intervention by nurse case managers includes assessment, advocacy, facilitation, teaching, support, collaborative problem solving, and evaluative follow-ups. Although this model needs further testing, its use with other populations may be helpful. Ahronheim (1997) suggests that advance directives (living wills, powers of attorney) are especially important for older women in poverty, whose voices in end-of-life decisions may be reduced. Exercise of autonomous choice is foundational to providing informed consent, which APNs must obtain from their patients. As Grace (2009) points out, an ethical standard for informing patients would include consideration of, "the patient's beliefs, values, and goals; the patient's ability to process information; and psychological, physiological, or environmental factors that might interfere with or facilitate processing of information" (p. 84). This subjective approach attends carefully to the patient's own circumstances. In the law, an objective, rather than a subjective approach typically would be used to assess the adequacy of the informed consent. An objective test would ascertain what a reasonable person would need to know. In either case, however, the patient would need to be capable of conveying a choice to the APN, and the APN could strive to accomplish both subjective and objective standards.

APN Autonomy

For the professional roles to evolve, APNs must experience autonomy in their judgments and practice. Ethical conflicts in practice have been found to decrease NPs' perceived autonomy (Ulrich & Soeken, 2005). Researchers have also found that NPs are concerned about ethical conflicts between the needs of patients and the requirements of managed care organizations (Butz, Redman, Fry, & Kolodner, 1998; Ulrich & Soeken, 2003). Also, conflicts of interest may hamper autonomy, for example, promotions of pharmaceuticals (Crigger, 2005). Ethical distress also stems from barriers APNs experience to the provision of ethical practice, such as the American Nurses Association's (ANA) unsuccessful effort to build the definition of a collaborative relationship with medicine in the mid-1990s. Although ANA and American Medical Association (AMA) representatives developed a definition of collaboration and ANA then passed a resolution in support of it, AMA has not yet passed a similar resolution (Giambarco, 2009). To face these challenges to their ethical integrity, APNs must reflect on their own values, allowing for serious, considered attention to the source of ethical conflict, and then work with others who share similar concerns toward resolution. In some of these situations, law can serve as an ally to APNs who seek change in regulations related to managed care organizations, the pharmaceutical industry, the definition of collaboration, and other areas of concern.

Choice and Finance

Choices made by patients and health care providers assume the existence of personal power to accomplish one's goals, and financial well-being is one form of power. Current estimates are that half of U.S. workers have inadequate pensions or savings for retirement (AARP, 2007a). As Parker and Thorslund (2007) note, the prevalence of health care problems increases as people age due to costs involved for health and social services and potentially long-term care. As baby boomers retire, pressure will be placed on government to provide adequate health care and other social services. If these supports are unavailable, poverty and its sequela will result. Current health reform efforts hope to address these financial realities. Poverty and poor health are correlated, according to Calero (2006). Likewise, poverty and mortality rates are correlated (the more poverty, the higher the mortality rates) (Sanchez & Albala, 2004). Without adequate financial support, persons are at risk in terms of health and social well-being. Wilson, Rogers, Chang, and Safran (2005) have found that cost-related medication skipping is associated with poverty among other variables, including poor health and relationship with one's physician. These health outcomes raise the criticism that current policy choices are resulting in poor health outcomes (consequentialism).

By way of example of the demographic changes that affect APN practice, Diczfalusy and Benagiano (1997) point to the expected increase in the percentage of the world population, including the United States, that is elderly—from 5.1% in 1950 to 8.8% in 2020—and note that most of the elderly are women and will have needs for social, economic, and health services that countries will be hard pressed to provide. Golant (2003) points out that for elderly persons, mostly women, who are cognitively and/or physically impaired, rental housing and needed community services are beyond reach economically. Older women also face discrimination, ageism, and loneliness, in addition to poverty (Sanchez-Salgado, 1998). Ahronheim (1997) also notes that older women in poverty are at risk for undertreatment of pain when they are terminally ill. Similarly, Howe (2006) notes that older persons may suffer emotional, as well as physical, pain, especially those with cognitive decline who face feelings of agitation, aggression, fear, depression, obsessions, or compulsions. When elderly must be placed in nursing homes, their autonomy is compromised in this institutional setting (Lidz, Fischer, & Arnold, 1992). Economic deprivation is also a form of injustice (deontology), but also means a lack of caring (ethic of care) or compassion (virtue ethics) for older persons. Individual choice becomes compromised in these situations of deprivation and threatens one's ability to behave autonomously.

JUSTICE AND VULNERABLE POPULATIONS

Justice means the fair and equitable treatment of others. As Butts and Rich (2008) state, "Justice as a principle in health care ethics refers to fairness, treating people equally and without prejudice, and the equitable distribution of benefits and burdens" (p. 48). One's effective personal, professional agency probably is not enough to deal with large-scale problems of poverty. Public policy change effected in law needs to accompany effective self-advocacy. As Wilson, Rogers, Chang, and Safran (2005) suggest, physicians should be aware of the risk factors associated with cost-related medication skipping (poverty and poor health), and discuss directly with their patients the financial problems patients may have paying for prescription medications and other treatments. As Calero (2006) says, poverty must be ended so that human dignity, universal rights, justice, enlightenment, and solidarity will exist among people. There is evidence that poverty predicts depression (Belle & Doucet, 2003). To bring about the policy change necessary to achieve equity for those in poverty, research outlining the realities throughout the world is necessary. Certain vulnerable groups, such as the elderly, women, ethnic minorities, and the poor, are sometimes excluded from research protocols (Larson, 1994). The World Health Organization's Commission on Social Determinants of Health collects pertinent evidence and recommends policy change to improve the health of vulnerable populations (Marmot, 2005). This data is critical to convincing lawmakers that change is necessary and that health is a vital factor in the well-being of the elderly and other vulnerable groups.

As Coburn (2004) avers, the structure of the political system of a country creates health consequences; in other words, countries with neo-liberal political policies that promote business progress in the global economy have more poverty and poorer health than social democratic countries. So if societies and organized health care organizations want to improve health, they will need to promote revolutionary change in the global marketplace and in evolving global political networks. And changes of social structures within societies must also be considered. For instance, Richardson (1999) points out that older women who retire face more family obligations, such as caregiving, than do men, and thus a realignment of caregiving responsibilities may be necessary so that older women's well-being and emancipation are achieved. In addition, political groups, such as organized labor, can help challenge the status quo to reduce the severe impact of poverty on working poor and retirees who become poor over time.

Societal and policy choices to assist or resist helping persons who become or are impoverished must consider the needs of others in the population, including children and people of all ages with disabilities that reduce their ability to achieve economic strength. Many authors have debated generational equity between young and old (Callahan, 1992; Kingson & Williamson, 1993; Minkler, 1986; Quadagno, 1990), and suggest that the resources of the country must be allocated in a fair fashion. They point out, for instance, that older people should not be grouped together as "wealthy" who benefit at the expense of children, but rather that consideration should be made of the wealth of specific individuals (means testing). This policy issue has direct and immediate impact on older persons who are poor, and their voices should be heard as these policy choices are made. Yet these individuals are often the least likely to be able to voice their concerns, and need others to act on their behalf. APNs can voice the concerns of the people in poverty whom they serve either through professional organizations or individual advocacy. For instance, they can work with the American Association of Retired Persons (AARP), which is building its powerbase in its "Divided We Fail" campaign to accomplish several goals, including:

1. Access to affordable and quality health care, including prescriptions
2. Upfront and understandable explanations of health care costs so people know what they are paying for

3. A less wasteful health care system
4. Affordable long-term care so people can remain in their homes and communities
5. A strong Social Security system for the next generations, without raising the national debt
6. Availability of tools and clear information to help manage finances and savings (AARP, 2007b).

SOURCES OF ETHICAL CONFLICT

In either providing patient care or advocating for policies that will increase the visibility of the problems faced by their patients, APNs find that issues of justice and fairness appear. Even in their own educational preparation, justice concerns emerge in their access to educational programs. NP programs should be accessible to all who are qualified regardless of income, but currently are not (Stark, Nair, & Omi, 1999). Several areas of patient-related ethical conflicts for NPs have been identified, including patient access to care, end-of-life decisions, beginning-of-life decisions, adolescent decision making, refusal of treatment, privacy, and violence.

Access to Care

One source of moral distress is difficulty accessing care because of transportation problems and reimbursement rules (Godfrey & Smith, 2002). This refers to the patient's health or social network limitations that pose problems in the ability to get to the office for care, and to complex Medicaid reimbursement rules such as the 1-year wait time rule for Pap smears, which prohibits women from obtaining a Pap smear during a postpartum visit. Some NPs felt the need to manipulate the system to obtain what the patient needed. In this situation, the NP's integrity is compromised, while her compassionate, beneficent response is served. Thus, two virtues are at odds as these NPs attempt to deal with the legal requirement.

End of Life

End-of-life care poses challenges for the APN, from questions of assistance in achieving a peaceful death to advanced planning for death. A study by Rabetoy and Bair (2007) demonstrated that few nephrology nurses and nephrology NPs had knowledge of the evidence-based clinical practice guideline for initiation and withdrawal of dialysis that had been released in 2000, and few had attended workshops to acquaint themselves with the guideline. They suggest that these nurses need to, "increase their awareness, knowledge, and possibly their comfort level with difficult, ethical patient care situations" (p. 606). Demarest (2004) points out roles that NPs can play in end-of-life care, similar to what physicians are encouraged to do: communication with the family, encouragement of advanced planning, supporting home care options, expressing empathy for the family, and dealing with their grief. In terms of assisted suicide, Hall (1996) points out that in states in which assisted suicide is legal, NPs who prescribe might be asked to prescribe lethal drugs to help patients die. She argues against the NPs choosing this path, which although legal in these jurisdictions, would violate ethical standards. As an evolving area of policy that is much in dispute, APNs should acquaint themselves with the law in their jurisdictions and position statements from professional organizations. Using self-reflection, APNs need to consider their own stances and be prepared to share their views in professional and policy arenas. APNs are also well positioned to discuss advance directives with patients and their families, so that the patient's preferences are known and expressed well before death (Schlenk, 1997). As she points out, advance planning for dying falls within the commitment that APNs have to primary prevention. Roessel (2007) echoes this call for NPs to discuss advance directives with patients so that they know what the patient wants, and can then decide their best role with the patient and family.

Beginning of Life

Ethical challenges are also found at the beginning of life, when vulnerable newborns need important health care decisions made on their behalf. Settle (2009) points out that neonatal nurse practitioners (NNPs) face ethical dilemmas that arise when family members and other staff disagree on actions to be taken for the newborn. Furthermore, she points out that legal ambiguities exist at the "margins of viability" (p. 198). She suggests regular interdisciplinary ethics rounds in which the decision makers communicate their viewpoints and seek consensus in their decisions.

Adolescents

Decisions made by adolescents also create concerns for APNs. Connolly (2001) points out the dilemma faced by the APN when girls under age

16 ask for contraceptives. Only 36 states allow contraceptives to be provided for adolescents without parental consent (Gaylord, 2009). As with assisted suicide, legal and ethical stances may be in conflict, causing the APN angst. Similarly, APNs in mental health practice with adolescents may practice in states that allow mentally ill adolescents to consent to treatment in the absence of their parents' consent. Roberson (2007a) points out the importance of research to understand the impact of these laws on treatment outcomes. In his dissertation research, he found that adolescents and their families preferred a collaborative role in making the decisions about mental health treatment (Roberson, 2007b). Even among adult mental health patients, a question of the adequacy of consent to treatment arises due to the "clouded judgment" of the patient, which "in turn renders voluntary informed decision-making difficult, if not impossible" (Grace & Terreri, 2009, p. 324). For this reason, 20 states have passed legislation authorizing the use of psychiatric advance directives, legal documents that allow a psychiatric patient to state a treatment preference for future mental health interventions, as well as a proxy if they lose the capacity to consent to treatment (Swanson, Swartz, Ferron, Elbogen, & Van Dorn, 2006). Similar approaches have been taken in European countries, as well (Henderson, Swanson, Szmukler, Thornicroft, & Zinkler, 2008).

Refusal of Treatment

In a study by Laabs (2005), she found that the most frequent ethical issue encountered in the practice of NPs was patient refusal of treatment. She speculates that NPs struggle with a conflict between autonomy and beneficence, which underlies many of the ethical conflicts they experience. When parents refuse vaccines for their children, for instance, APNs will be caught in a serious dilemma, as is society, which must enact laws that protect the community. Thus far, as Gaylord (2009) points out, in all states and nationally, vaccinations have not been mandated. To resolve these dilemmas, she suggests use of an ethic-of-care approach to ensure that the supportive relationships needed by patients and families are intact. Another area of refusal of care is the patient's execution of a Do Not Resuscitate (DNR) order. Conflicts exist most specifically in surgical situations in which the question of suspension of the DNR arises. Several anesthesia organizations, including the American Association of Nurse Anesthetists, have taken an opportunity to develop positions in opposition to automatic suspension of DNRs during surgery. Instead, they recommend an open discussion with the patient or the patient's proxy before the surgery to come to an agreement about what procedures, if any, will be suspended (Sheedy, 2009).

Privacy and Confidentiality

Privacy and confidentiality issues also arise in APN practice. Privacy refers to the right to limit access of others to one's personal information, and confidentiality prevents release of personal information to others (Beauchamp & Childress, 2009). In a study of primary care APNs and their patients, researchers found several APN concerns:

1. breaches in privacy occurring through carelessness
2. concern about over-regulation
3. establishment of trust between provider and patient
4. overlap between providers and patients
5. patients' control of information
6. situations involving sensitive information
7. electronic data storage and transmission
8. mandated information reporting
9. situations with adolescents, who present special problems (Deshefy-Longhi, Dixon, Olsen, & Grey, 2004, p. 387).

When patient and APN concerns were compared, APNs were found to be more concerned with carelessness, and patients more worried about disclosures of research information (Olsen, Dixon, Grey, Deshefy-Longhi, & Demarest, 2005). Butz, Redman, Fry, and Kolodner (1998) also found concerns with confidentiality in their study of certified pediatric nurse practitioners (PNPs). The most common concern of these PNPs was requests from parents for sexual information about their adolescent children who were either sexually active or pregnant. Standards for privacy and confidentiality come from ethics sources in codes of ethics, and the law in statutes such as the Health Insurance Portability and Accountability Act of 1996 (HIPAA), a series of federal acts found in Titles 18, 29, and 42 of the United States Code. Similar privacy problems may appear with genetic testing, as this becomes more common (Havens & Kovner, 1997). APNs are also concerned about breaking confidentiality when the law requires certain activities to be reported, such as child abuse and threats of violence made by psychiatric mental health patients.

Violence

In situations of violence such as child abuse, APNs may wonder what and when to report incidences of neglect or abuse. As Butz, Redman,

Fry, and Kolodner (1998) report, PNPs struggle with this decision because of the implications for family relationships, questions of future care of the child, and degree and types of evidence that must be reported. In women's health care, an issue of power imbalances between women and men in our society sometimes leads to difficulty in discerning the concerns of women who feel powerless (Smith, 2009). She points out that domestic violence, maternal–fetal conflict, and infertility treatment raise these concerns for APNs, and suggests a "feminist ethic of care" (p. 277), wherein an understanding of the unique aspects of the individual woman becomes apparent in authentic dialogue with the APN.

Consequences of Ethical Conflict

As Godfrey and Smith (2002) point out, sustained and intense ethical conflicts can lead to moral fatigue, described by Taylor (2002) as a "weariness" resulting from a "loss of sensitivity" to ongoing ethical challenges (p. 41). Corley (2002) proposes a theory and research agenda to understand moral distress, which results from the failure to complete goals that the nurse has set. Conscience clauses that allow the APN to refuse care to certain patients on the basis of religious objections can be exercised by APNs in many states, but raise access-to-care problems for patients seeking certain medications or abortions (Wilson, 2008).

APN SELF-REFLECTIONS AND ACTIONS

Motivations of APNs who serve as advocates for their patients stem from various ethical vantage points, and should be examined self-reflectively as interventions are developed and evaluated. From a deontological perspective, principles such as justice, beneficence, and autonomy are served by advocating for more resources for the poor and vulnerable. From a teleological view, APNs can work for ends such as policy options that result in improved health care and successful social and economic skills. APNs can recognize their own feelings (sympathy and empathy) for vulnerable patients as the ethic of care prescribes, and their character traits and those of their clients as virtue ethics expects. On the broader scale, nurses may act from concern about the community's health (communitarianism) and with assessments that distinguish characteristics of each case (casuistry). Any or all of these ethical benchmarks may be selected by nurses to determine actions that are appropriate for use with their patients, families, and communities.

Rittenbach (2005) found the participant NPs in her study relied half of the time on the ethic of care; a combination of justice and care-based approaches were also used by these NPs to resolve ethical dilemmas. Shirey (2007) suggests personal assessment by Clinical Nurse Specialists (CNSs) of their moral competence, which she defines as, "doing the right thing," following the contemplation of the nature of right action consistent with one's values. In a study of the way that NPs handle moral problems to maintain their integrity, Laabs (2007) found that they used a four-stage process:

1. Encountering a conflict situation
2. Drawing a line concerning what the NP was and was not willing to do in the situation
3. Finding a way to meet the needs of the patient without crossing the line
4. Evaluating one's actions in terms of how well the NP's integrity had been maintained (Laabs, p. 799).

If the NP could not maintain integrity (stage four), moral distress resulted, and the NP would either avoid the problem, compensate for his or her action, or convince himself or herself that the proper action had been taken. Critical to the process is a consideration of the context in which care is delivered, such as agency policies and budgetary or legal constraints (Kalb & O'Connor-Von, 2007; Laabs, 2007; Peterson & Potter, 2004; Ulrich & Soeken, 2003).

Contemplation of one's own values and nursing codes of ethics are valuable sources of information. Peterson and Potter (2004) argue for development of a code of ethics for the roles of NPs that includes both nursing and medical standards that are distinct from codes of ethics for all nurses, such as that of the ANA (ANA, 2001) or the International Council of Nurses (International Council of Nurses, 2009). Two specialty areas have their own codes of ethics: certified nurse midwives (ACNM, 2009) and certified registered nurse anesthetists (AANA, 2009). (See Table 2.1 for a comparison of ethical tenets from several nursing codes of ethics.) Because there are variations among the codes, the APN must consider the specific focus of their practice, legal requirements in their jurisdictions, and their own sense of integrity in deciding the actions to take and potential consequences of these actions.

Formal ethics programs would be useful in helping APNs to clarify and then reduce conflicts within their work environments (Butz, Redman, Fry, & Kolodner, 1998; Ulrich & Soeken, 2003, 2005). Some studies have shown the need for ethics education for APNs to help them understand privacy and confidentiality (Deshefy-Longhi, Dixon,

Table 2.1

CODES OF ETHICS

ETHICAL STANDARD	PROPOSED CODE (PETERSON & POTTER, 2004)	ANA CODE (2001)	ICN CODE (2006)	ACNM CODE (2005)	AANA CODE (2005)
Competent care	X	X	X	X	X
Compassion	X	X		X	
Confidentiality/privacy	X	X	X	X	X
Respect for persons	X	X	X	X	X
Responsibility to patients (family, group, community)	X	X	X	X	X
Access of care to all	X	X	X	X	X
Collaboration with other health care providers	X	X	X	X	X
Legal accountability	X	X		X	X
Advocacy for patients' rights	X	X		X	X
Professional self-development	X	X	X	X	X
Education of public	X	X		X	
Attentive to environment of care	X	X	X	X	X
Ethical business practices		X		X	X
Truthful endorsement of products/services				X	X
Research integrity		X	X	X	X
Maintain integrity of profession		X		X	
Protect from harmful acts of others		X	X	X	X
Support education of students		X	X	X	
Maintain own health and integrity		X	X	X	X
Policy development		X		X	X
Maintain professional boundaries		X		X	X
Conscientious objection		X		X	X

Olsen, & Grey, 2004), and to understand respect for human dignity (Kalb & O'Connor-Von (2007). Likewise, use of ethics committees or ethics consults to discuss and resolve ethical conflicts is a valuable resource to use if available to the APN (Grace, 2009). However, as Butz and colleagues (1998) reported in their study of PNPs, few conflicts were referred to an ethics committee. If a more powerful means of resolving ethical disputes is needed, Schlairet (2009) suggests use of bioethics mediation, a process using dispute resolution skills to reach a mutually agreed-upon solution.

Whatever routes are chosen by APNs to improve the lives of their patients, attention to their own internal ethical motivations will result in greater self-satisfaction (sense of integrity) for the nurse, and potentially greater effectiveness in policy choices and health outcomes. Policy action developed by nursing organizations acting in conjunction with consumer groups is most likely to be effective in making needed change. And the voices of individual patients who testify before policymaking committees will provide powerful support for change. As the mentally ill have become adept at testifying publicly, so can other groups of patients with support from those who care deeply about their well-being, such as APNs. Although the law is as Butz and colleagues (1998, p. 189) point out, "a blunt instrument," shaping the law carefully with the appropriate tool will create a more flexible and responsive instrument to meet the needs of diverse populations of APNs and those they serve.

SUMMARY

APNs alone, or in conjunction with influential groups representing the interests of patients, families, and communities, create a powerful force to instigate needed health care reform and other policy changes. APNs are advocates for their patients, and can use ethics consultations or bioethics mediation strategies to resolve conflicts in clinical situations (Grace, 2009; Schlairet, 2009). Whether APNs are motivated by a sense of justice, caring, duty, evidence-based interventions, or compelling details, their actions taken to improve the status of patients and families will improve society as a whole. With improved care of patients, each member of society can look forward to a healthful life. APNs are well positioned to improve the physical, mental, and moral health of clients, families, and their communities, thus strengthening their own voices as advocates for change.

KEY POINTS

1. Apologies for error by providers reduce costly litigation and reflect a compassionate ethical base.
2. Threats to the autonomy of patients and APNs require self-reflection to know one's true values prior to responding to the threat.
3. APNs can advocate for patients in poverty through professional organizations or, individually, in patient care situations.
4. Many conflicts faced by APNs involve the tension between autonomy and beneficence.
5. Ethics education, use of ethics committees, and bioethics mediation will help APNs to resolve the ethical conflicts they face.

REFERENCES

AARP. (2007a). Divided we fail. *AARP Bulletin, 48*(2), 3–5.
AARP. (2007b). AARP needs you. *AARP: The Magazine, 50*(3b), 44.
Ahronheim, J. C. (1997). End-of-life issues for very elderly women: Incurable and terminal illness. *Journal of the American Medical Women's Association, 52*(3), 147–151.
American Association of Nurse Anesthetists (AANA). (2005). *Code of ethics for the certified registered nurse anesthetist.* Retrieved July 8, 2008, from http://www.aana. com/resources.aspx?ucNavMenu_TSMenuTargetID=51&ucNavMenu_TSMenuTarg etType=4&ucNavMenu_TSMenuID=6&id=665
American College of Nurse Midwives (ACNM). (2005). *Code of ethics with explanatory statements.* American College of Nurse-Midwives. Retrieved April 19, 2010, from http://www.midwife.org/siteFiles/education/CodeOfEthicswithExplan atoryStatements2005.pdf
American Nurses Association (ANA). (2001). *Code of ethics for nurses with interpretive statements.* Washington, DC: Author.
Beauchamp, T. L., & Childress, J. F. (2009). *Principles of biomedical ethics* (6th ed.). New York: Oxford University Press.
Belle, D., & Doucet, J. (2003). Poverty, inequality, and discrimination as sources of depression among U.S. women. *Psychology of Women Quarterly, 27*(2), 101–113.
Blacksher, E. (2002). On being poor and feeling poor: Low socioeconomic status and the moral self. *Theoretical Medicine, 23*(6), 455–470.
Butts, J. B., & Rich, K. L. (2008). *Nursing ethics across the curriculum and into practice* (2nd ed.). Boston: Jones and Bartlett.
Butz, A. M., Redman, B. K., Fry, S. T., & Kolodner, K. (1998). Ethical conflicts experienced by certified pediatric nurse practitioner in ambulatory settings. *Journal of Pediatric Health Care, 12*(4), 183–190.
Calero, J. (2006). Demographic changes and health management. *Anales de Law Real Academia Nacional de Medicina, 123*(1), 153–174.

Callahan, D. (1992). Reforming the health care system for children and the elderly to balance cure and care. *Academic Medicine, 67*(4), 219–222.

Coburn, D. (2004). Beyond the income inequality hypothesis: Class, neo-liberalism, and health inequalities. *Social Science & Medicine, 58*(1), 41–56.

Connolly, J. (2001). Contraception and the under 16's—Legal and ethical implications for the advanced nurse practitioner. In K. Bartter (Ed.), *Ethical issues in advanced nursing practice.* Oxford, UK: Butterworth-Heinemann.

Corley, M. C. (2002). Nurse moral distress: A proposed theory and research agenda. *Nursing Ethics, 9*(6), 636–650.

Crigger, N. L. (2005). Pharmaceutical promotions and conflict of interest in nurse practitioners' decision making: The undiscovered country. *Journal of the American Academy of Nurse Practitioners, 17*(6), 207–212.

Demarest, P. (2004). The role of nurse practitioners in end-of-life care. *Journal of the American Medical Association, 291*(20), 2432.

Deshefy-Longhi, T., Dixon, J. K., Olsen, D., & Grey, M. (2004). Privacy and confidentiality issues in primary care: Views of advanced practice nurses and their patients. *Nursing Ethics, 11*(4), 378–393.

Diczfalusy, E., & Benagiano, G. (1997). Women and the third and fourth age. *Journal of International Gyneacology and Obstetrics, 58*(1), 177–188.

Gaylord, N. (2009). Nursing ethics and advanced practice: Children and adolescents. In P. J. Grace (Ed.), *Nursing ethics and professional responsibility in advanced practice* (pp. 221–245). Boston: Jones and Bartlett.

Giambarco, D. (2009). Collaborative relationships—Promoting patient good. In P. J. Grace (Ed.), *Nursing ethics and professional responsibility in advanced practice* (pp. 135–152). Boston: Jones and Bartlett.

Godfrey, N., & Smith, K. (2002). Moral distress and the nurse practitioner. *Journal of Clinical Ethics, 13*(4), 330–336.

Goering, L. (2007, April 15). India's elderly suffer as younger generations look the other way. *News & Observer,* p. 16A.

Golant, S. M. (2003). Political and organizational barriers to satisfying low-income U.S. seniors' need for affordable rental housing with supportive services. *Journal of Aging and Social Policy, 15*(4), 21–48.

Grace, P. J. (2009). *Nursing ethics and professional responsibility in advanced practice.* Boston: Jones and Bartlett.

Grace, P. J., & Terreri, P. A. (2009). Nursing ethics and advanced practice: Psychiatric and mental health issues. In P. J. Grace (Ed.), *Nursing ethics and professional responsibility in advanced practice* (pp. 317–338). Boston: Jones and Bartlett.

Hall, J. (1996). Assisted suicide: Nurse practitioners as providers? *Nurse Practitioner, 21*(10), 63–66, 71.

Havens, D. M., & Kovner, R. (1997). Genetic testing: How it is transforming the role of health professionals and the implications for pediatric nurse practitioners. *Journal of Pediatric Health Care, 11*(4), 193–197.

Henderson, C., Swanson, J. W., Szmukler, G., Thornicroft, G., & Zinkler, M. (2008). A typology of advance statements in mental health care. *Psychiatric Services, 59*, 63–71.

Howe, E. G. (2006). Do we undervalue feelings in patients who are cognitively impaired? *Journal of Clinical Ethics, 17*(4), 291–301.

International Council of Nurses. (2006). *The ICN code of ethics for nurses.* Retrieved April 19, 2010, from http://www.icn.ch/icncode.pdf

Kalb, K. A., & O'Connor-Von, S. (2007). Ethics education in advanced practice nursing: Respect for human dignity. *Nursing Education Perspectives, 28*(4), 196–202.

Kingson, E. R., & Williamson, J. B. (1993). The generational equity debate: A progressive framing of a conservative issue. *Journal of Aging and Social Policy, 5*(3), 31–53.

Laabs, C. A. (2005). Moral problems and distress among nurse practitioners in primary care. *Journal of the American Academy of Nurse Practitioners, 17*(2), 76–84.

Laabs, C. A. (2007). Primary care nurse practitioners' integrity when faced with moral conflict. *Nursing Ethics, 14*(6), 795–809.

Lange, A. J., & Jakubowski, P. (1976). *Responsible assertive behavior: Cognitive/behavioral procedures for trainers.* Champaign, IL: Research Press.

Larson, E. (1994). Exclusion of certain groups from clinical research. *Image: A Journal of Nursing Scholarship, 26*(3), 185–190.

Lidz, C. W., Fischer, L., & Arnold, R. M. (1992). *The erosion of autonomy in long-term care.* New York: Oxford University Press.

Maliski, S. L., Clerkin, B., & Litwin, M. S. (2004). Describing a nurse case manager intervention to empower low-income men with prostate cancer. *Oncology Nursing Forum, 31*(1), 57–64.

Marmot, M. (2005). Social determinants of health inequities. *Lancet, 365*(9464), 1005–1006.

Meadows, R. (2007). Beyond caring. *Nursing Administration Quarterly, 31*(2), 158–161.

Minkler, M. (1986). "Generational equity" and the new victim blaming: An emerging public policy issue. *International Journal of Health Services, 16*(4), 539–551.

Minow, M. (1990). *Making all the difference: Inclusion, exclusion, and American law.* Ithaca, NY: Cornell University Press.

Olsen, D. P., Dixon, J. K., Grey, M., Deshefy-Longhi, T., & Demarest, J. (2005). Privacy concerns of patients and nurse practitioners in primary care—An APRNet study. *Journal of the American Academy of Nurse Practitioners, 17*(12), 527–534.

Parker, M. G., & Thorslund, M. (2007). Health trends in the elderly population: Getting better and getting worse. *The Gerontologist, 47*(2), 150–158.

Peterson, M., & Potter, R. L. (2004). A proposal for a code of ethics for nurse practitioners. *Journal of the American Academy of Nurse Practitioners, 16*(3), 116–124.

Quadagno, J. (1990). Generational equity and the politics of the welfare state. *International Journal of Health Services, 20*(4), 631–649.

Rabetoy, C. P., & Bair, B. C. (2007). Nephrology nurses' perspectives on difficult ethical issues and practice guideline for shared decision making. *Nephrology Nursing Journal, 34*(6), 599–606, 629.

Richardson, V. E. (1999). Women and retirement. *Journal of Women and Aging, 11*(2–3), 49–66.

Rittenbach, T. H. (2005). *A framework of moral reasoning for nurse practitioners.* Unpublished doctoral dissertation, University of Minnesota, Minneapolis.

Roberson, A. J. (2007a). Adolescent informed consent: Ethics, law, and theory to guide policy and nursing research. *Journal of Nursing Law, 11*(4), 191–196.

Roberson, A. J. (2007b). *The experiences of adolescents consenting to psychiatric mental health treatment.* Unpublished doctoral dissertation, University of North Carolina at Chapel Hill.

Roessel, L. L. (2007). Protect your patients' rights with advance directives. *Nurse Practitioner: The American Journal of Primary Health Care, 32*(8), 38–39, 41–43.

Sack, K. (2008, May 18). More docs admit to errors: They find integrity in honest regret. *News & Observer,* p. 6A.

Sanchez, H., & Albala, C. (2004). Inequalities in health: Adult mortality in communities of metropolitan Santiago. *Revista Medica de Chile, 132*(4), 453–460.

Sanchez-Salgado, C. D. (1998). Feminization of old age in Puerto Rico. *Puerto Rico Health Science Journal, 17*(1), 49–53.

Schlairet, M. C. (2009). Bioethics mediation: The role and importance of nursing advocacy. *Nursing Outlook, 57*(4), 185–193.

Schlenk, J. S. (1997). Advance directives: Role of nurse practitioners. *Journal of the American Academy of Nurse Practitioners, 9*(7), 317–321.

Settle, P. D. (2009). Nursing ethics and advanced practice: Neonatal issues. In P. J. Grace (Ed.), *Nursing ethics and professional responsibility in advanced practice* (pp. 191–219). Boston: Jones and Bartlett.

Sheedy, G. (2009). Nursing ethics and nurse anesthesia practice. In P. J. Grace (Ed.), *Nursing ethics and professional responsibility in advanced practice* (pp. 339–381). Boston: Jones and Bartlett.

Shirey, M. (2007). Moral intelligence for the leader and entrepreneur. *Clinical Nurse Specialist: A Journal for Advanced Nursing Practice, 21*(2), 71–73.

Smith, K. T. (2009). Nursing ethics and advanced practice: Women's health. In P. J. Grace (Ed.), *Nursing ethics and professional responsibility in advanced practice* (pp. 247–280). Boston: Jones and Bartlett.

Stark, R., Nair, N., & Omi, S. (1999). Nurse practitioners in developing countries: Some ethical considerations. *Nursing Ethics, 6*(4), 273–277.

Swanson, J., Swartz, M., Ferron, J., Elbogen, E., & Van Dorn, R. (2006). Psychiatric advance directives among public mental health consumers in five U.S. cities: Prevalence, demand, and correlates. *Journal of the American Academy of Psychiatry and the Law, 34*(1), 43–57.

Taylor, S. (2002). Moral fatigue—A nursing perspective. *Bioethics Forum, 18*(1–2), 37–43.

Ulrich, C. M., & Soeken, K. L. (2003). Ethical conflict associated with managed care: Views of nurse practitioners. *Nursing Research, 52*(3), 168–175.

Ulrich, C. M., & Soeken, K. L. (2005). A path analytic model of ethical conflict in practice and autonomy in a sample of nurse practitioners. *Nursing Ethics, 12*(3), 305–316.

Wilson, I. B., Rogers, W. H., Chang, H., & Safran, D. G. (2005). Cost-related skipping of medications and other treatments among Medicare beneficiaries between 1998 and 2000. Results of a national study. *Journal of General Internal Medicine, 8,* 715–720.

Wilson, R. F. (2008). The limits of conscience: Moral clashes over deeply divisive healthcare procedures. *American Journal of Law & Medicine, 34*(1), 41–63.

3

Policy Changes Affecting Advanced Practice

DIANE KJERVIK

Political activism has always been at the heart of advanced practice nursing.

—*J. Pulcini and M. A. Hart*

To move beyond entry-level practice, advanced practice nurses (APNs) have advocated steadily for legislative and regulatory changes in rules for practice arrangements to allow them to prescribe, diagnose, and treat patients. These policy changes have led to increasing independence from physicians and the medical model, and toward development of nursing practice models that address more complex patient, family, community, and institutional components. In defining "policy," Mason, Leavitt, and Chafee (2007) point out that, "policy encompasses the choices that a society, segment of society, or organization makes regarding its goals and priorities and the ways it allocates its resources to attain those goals" (p. 3). Clearly, nursing, as a segment of society, has made a choice of goals and use of resources in support of its goal to build advanced nursing practice.

When the choices are made by public entities, such as legislatures or courts, public policy results, and is considered public because its application affects all of the persons served by the legal body. If private entities, such as professional organizations or privately run agencies, are involved, private policy is the result, and its application is only to the organization and members involved. This chapter examines some of the choices nursing has made to develop advanced practice, including a proposed regulatory model for advanced practice registered nurses (APRNs), whistleblowing, billing issues, retail clinics, the Doctor of Nursing Practice (DNP) degree, and opportunities for APNs in the current health care reform climate.

REGULATORY MODELS FOR ADVANCED PRACTICE REGISTERED NURSES

Recently, the National Council of State Boards of Nursing, working with advanced practice leaders, published a statement of consensus about regulation of APNs (National Council of State Boards of Nursing [NCSBN], 2008). Twenty-three organizations developed the consensus statement after working together from 2004 to 2008 (Stanley, 2009). To develop a synchronized approach to education, accreditation, licensure, and certification requirements, the consensus statement addressed all four of these categories so that the practice goals of patient safety and increased access to the skills of APRNs could be achieved. APRNs include certified registered nurse anesthetists (CRNAs), certified nurse midwives (CNMs), clinical nurse specialists (CNSs), and certified nurse practitioners (NPs). The lack of uniformity from one state to another led to confusion in the public about APN roles (Stanley, 2009). Because state regulations vary for these advanced practice roles, the consensus statement offers an approach that will reduce these variations, resulting in easier movement of the APRN from one state to another and greater access for patients to APRN services (NCSBN, 2008). Thus, consumers, health care agencies, and policymakers, as well as APRNs, will have clearer understanding of APRN roles and responsibilities.

The proposed model includes detailed definitions of APRNs, describing their responsibilities for "health promotion and the assessment, diagnosis, and management of patient problems, which includes the use and prescription of pharmacologic and non-pharmacologic interventions" (NCSBN, 2008, p. 6). As Rozga (2009) points out, "prescription power is the most significant component of the RHC (retail health clinic) business model" (p. 219). In all probability, prescriptive authority provides APNs bargaining power with many other employers, in addition to a greater ability to be in charge of their own private practices.

Currently, there are state-by-state variations in prescriptive authority that this model seeks to standardize. The model also proposes licensure and a legally protected title at the advanced practice level. As Safriet (2002) points out, scopes of practice, "legislatively-defined spheres of

activity within which various types of health care providers are authorized to practice" (p. 303), do not clearly link legal authority and clinical
ability. The consensus model does emphasize ability and links types of
abilities to legal recognition of titles. Licensure would be in one of the
four APRN roles within one of the specified population groups (family/
individual across the life span, adult/gerontology, neonatal, pediatrics,
women's health, psychiatric-mental health) (NCSBN, 2008). Interestingly, a foundational requirement of every board of nursing will be
to "license APRNs as independent practitioners with no regulatory
requirements for collaboration, direction or supervision" (NCSBN,
2008, p. 13). Also, APRNs are to be licensed solely by nursing boards
(Stanley, 2009). Further specialization will not appear on APRN licenses, but certification in specialties will be possible. A new specialty,
comprehensive care, developed at Columbia University for APRNs with
DNP degrees, requires passing an exam that is "narrower in scope than
the three step exam that doctors take," but otherwise is similar to the
exam that MDs must take for licensure (Landro, 2008, p. D1). These
requirements for licensure and certification will meet resistence from
medical societies in some states. Some physician groups have expressed
concern that there will be a blurring of responsbilities between MDs
and APRNs, which will lead to public confusion (Landro, 2008).

Education of APRNs must include a graduate degree or postgraduate
certificate from an academic, accredited institution and passing a national certification exam. The consensus model does not specify doc-
toral-level graduate degrees such as the DNP, which has been
recommended by the American Association of Colleges of Nursing as
a requirement for APNs by 2015 (AACN, 2009). However, the consensus
statement does target 2015 for full implementation (Stanley, 2009).
When fully implemented, the unified model should provide greater
efficiency in admininstration and greater ease in collection of workforce
data (Stanley, 2009).

The consensus statement provides a policy aspiration for each state
and nursing organization. Consumer groups also have a stake in the
success of this plan, and nursing organizations will work closely to
gain adoption by legal authorities (legislatures, licensure boards, and
courts that will be asked to interpret the statutes, rules, and regulations).
Broadening the consensus beyond the nursing community will be essential to its success.

WHISTLEBLOWING

Although the American Nurses Association (ANA) Code of Ethics and
some state boards of nursing require nurses to report the unethical or

incompetent conduct of their colleagues, these requirements may not protect the nurse from action against his or her employment following his or her report of this conduct (Mason, Leavitt, & Chaffee, 2007). ANA's *Nursing World* reports that 20 states, as of July 2009, have enacted whistleblowing protections for health care providers (ANA, 2009). Only specific whistleblowing legislation stating that retaliation is prohibited will be capable of providing this protection. And criminal charges might also be filed, as happened in Texas in 2009 (Inglis, 2009). In this case, two nurses from a 25-bed hospital in west Texas reported allegedly substandard practice by a physician in the hospital. They were fired after filing an anonymous report with the Board of Medicine and included medical record numbers of the patients involved, but not their names.

The physician filed a harassment complaint against the nurses with the Sheriff's office, and the sheriff investigated details of the case, which led him to the names of the nurses. A grand jury then indicted them for misuse of official information (Barbee, 2009). Both the Texas Nursing and Medical Boards objected to the prosecution, as did the Texas Nurses Association and the ANA. Although this could be, as Inglis (2009) states, "a stunning display of good ol' boy idiocy and abuse of prosecutorial discretion," and unlikely to occur in any other jurisdiction in the United States, the fact that it could happen at all has sent shivers up the spines of other potential whistleblowers.

The ANA advocates for inclusion of whistleblowing protections in specific types of legislation, such as patient safety, patient bill of rights, health reform, and patient protection at the federal level, as well as provisions at the state level (Mason, Leavitt, & Chaffee, 2007). An example of specific whistleblowing legislation affecting APN practice is related to health care fraud. The False Claims Act (1982) allows for damages to be paid to the U.S. government for filing false Medicaid claims (fraudulent billing). Hannigan (2006) describes several types of billing problems: "upcoding" (p. 512), in which more services are billed than were actually provided, double-billing, billing for services performed by someone who was not credentialled to provide the service, and unbundling, in which services performed together are billed as separate events. The Stark II law (1998), a civil statute, prohibits referrals of Medicare patients to anyone or any legal entity that has a financial relationship with the provider. The Anti-kickback Statute (1994) is a criminal statute that prohibits financial inducements for referrals. Although some protections exist for whistleblowers, risk of losing employment still exists, according to Hannigan, (2006), who raises the question of whether to report this, and concludes that the APN should consider carefully the legal and practical ramifications of reporting billing and reimbursement fraud.

Practical considerations that Hannigan (2006) suggests be considered include whether the injustice is serious and well substantiated, ethically grounded, whether blowing the whistle will result in "more good than harm" (p. 515) to the patient, and whether the APN is willing to accept responsibility for the consequences of reporting. Consequences are often difficult to decipher, however, which means that consultation with a lawyer in the given state will be necessary prior to reporting. Consultation with the state board of nursing to ascertain its requirements and protections, if any, is also worth doing. Loss of employment, even for ethically correct reasons, may be too high a price for the APN to pay. If there is any way for a group or organization of APNs rather than a single APN to blow the whistle, this may result in less severe consequences to the APN.

APN COMPLIANCE WITH STATE LAW

State boards of nursing in some states have audited the records of NPs and their collaborating physicians, as reported by Buppert (2008). Alabama, North Carolina, and Virginia have audited records of NPs and physicians for compliance with protocols, specifying activities including treatments and drugs that may be prescribed by the NP, whether a collaborative agreement is in place, and whether the physician is on site, as is required by law. As Buppert (2008) points out, these audits might chill the willingness of physicians to hire NPs. On the other hand, she cautions that NPs might lose sight of state requirements if periodic audits are not required.

If the consensus statement for regulation of APRNs as proposed by the NCSBN (2008) becomes law in all states, APNs and physicians will be more aware of the legal requirements of them. Their understanding will not be altered by moving from one state to another, which not only will assist consumers to know what services can be expected, but also providers.

BILLING ISSUES

Reimbursement for services is vital to the health of APN practice. Federal, state, and private payers provide payment for these services, but with numerous gray areas in policy. As Buppert (2009) points out in referrring to billing for provider services in hospitals, "there is no single, government-produced document that NPs, physicians, and hospital adminstrators can refer to for clear direction on these matters" (Introduction, para. 4). Even definitions of coding categories for billing (*International Statistical Classification of Diseases-9* [*ICD-9*]; World Health Organization, 1977) for diagnoses and current procedural terminology for procedures are not always clear (Phillipsen, Setlow, & Jacob, 2008). As a result, APNs are encouraged to attend classes or receive consultation on coding for accuracy (Phillipsen, Setlow, & Jacob, 2008). Without accurate billing, the APN could have legal problems, including the potential loss of professional licensure.

Rickard (2009) points out the value of NPs and CNSs to health care practices, with specific focus on financial profit to the practice. She cautions, however, that practices need to become familiar with state and federal reimbursement regulations to avoid audits and claim denials. Health care attorneys will be an important factor in helping the practice to find ways to understand what is required. For instance, the distinctions between direct billing, "incident to" billing, and shared/split-visit billing for Medicare are critical to understand to maximize reimbursement for APN practice (Rickard, 2009).

The American Association of Nurse Attorneys (AANA, 2005) has issued a guidebook for APNs, which includes a discussion of ways the NPs can enroll to participate as a provider for Medicare, Medicaid, and other federal payers, as well as nongovernmental payers. Buppert (2005) has developed a detailed guide to billing practices for primary care providers to prevent legal problems through proper documentation and understanding of ongoing requirements.

APNs working in hospitals should be aware that some services, such as rounding and transfer orders, are not billable to Medicare (Buppert, 2009). And even though some states do not require a collaborative agreement with a physician, Medicare does (Buppert, 2009). So, APNs need to be well aware of the myriad rules, both state and federal, as well as from private third-party payers, that direct their care of patients.

RETAIL CLINICS

APNs are quite familiar with fighting their own battles for acceptance in health care circles, and have discovered that opportunities for partnerships with nonhealth care organizations result in achievement of goals important to both. Business arrangements to provide health care services to patrons of grocery stores, pharmacies in drug stores, or major stores such as Wal-Mart, have appeared as a result of public pressure for accessible, high-quality care at convenient locations (Hsu, 2008). NPs and physician's assistants (PAs) typically provide services in these clinics where wait times are short, no appointments are necessary, and the costs are lower than doctor's offices. Services provided are for uncomplicated primary care services, such as sore throats, colds, flu, immunizations, and allergies. These new venues for ANP practice have created controversy from medical groups, such as the American Medical Association, which "has raised issues regarding potential conflicts of interest, continuity of care, and the use of non-physician providers" (Hsu, 2008, p. 13).

From a strictly nursing malpractice perspective, NPs would be liable for the same standard of care and scope of practice in retail clinics as in other practice sites within their states, and thus, the stir about increased risk in retail is, according to Miller (2008), uncalled for. In fact, the American Academy of Nurse Practitioners (AANP) has published standards for NPs who practice in retail clinics (AANP, 2009). These standards include the expectation that NPs meet regulatory requirements, participate actively in the development and management of the business, that they assess and treat patients, including referral to others when necessary, and meet other professional expectations. However, corporate liability is another matter, and lawyers who represent retail clinics must attend to this, as well.

Legal challenges remain that must be resolved for this new type of health delivery model to be successful. The Convenient Care Association represents several of the national chains with retail clinics and "attempts to ease physician fears by promulgating national standards that promote high quality of care and a minimal competitive threat" (Rozga, 2009, p. 211). Both certificate of need (CON) and corporate practice of medicine (CPOM) requirements vary from state to state (Rozga, 2009). CONs are required of agencies wishing to establish business in the state, and CPOM laws specify requirements for businesses in terms of whether they may be physician-owned (Rozga, 2009). Also, conflicts of interest may exist in profit-generating referral arrangements that are prohibited by Stark II (1998) or Anti-kickback Laws (1994). Concerns also exist about a potential conflict of interest arising from the proximity of the practice to sales of drugs and supplies. The legal question is whether the relationship between the clinic and the pharmacy in the store is a proper business relationship (Hsu, 2008). From the consumer perspective, however, they can visit the clinic, and if they have to wait for a provider, they can shop, so they find the arrangement to be advantageous. Some clinics will lend a pager to the clients so that they can be notified when the provider is available (Hsu, 2008).

Physician concerns about quality of care meet face-to-face with the retail store's wish to offer this service to their customers, and thus, instead of NPs and PAs fighting the battles on their own, the retailers raise the arguments. When physician groups push for restrictive regulations on retail clinics, the retailers can argue that consumer access to care will be more limited (Hsu, 2008). When the physicians express concern that the doctor–patient relationship will be impaired by visits to a retail clinic, retailers can argue that the legal relationship between the NP and the physician will be formally documented in support of continuity of care (Hsu, 2008). Thus, the retail store venue for APN services shows rich promise of a win-win-win approach to the provision of health care services for the patient, NP, and the retailer. Whether physicians can impede or otherwise resist the competitive challenge is yet to be determined.

EVOLVING APN PRACTICE AND EDUCATIONAL REFORM

As APN practice evolves, new specialities appear. The Comprehensive Care specialty for APRNs was mentioned previously, but other possibilities exist for future development of specialties and subspecialties. For instance, Bowring-Lossock (2006) discusses the development of a new focus on forensic mental health nursing in England and Wales. This role serves the mentally ill offender, whereas in the United States, the primary focus of forensic nursing is on the victim of crime. This role in the United Kingdom involves obtaining specialty knowledge beyond the basic level of education in psychiatric nursing, but does not require an advanced degree. In this sense, the preparation for the forensic mental health nurse role would be similar to that of the sexual assault nurse examiner (SANE) in the United States. Other subspecialties that are evolving are palliative care, hospitalist, emergency preparedness, and health care genetics (National Organization of Nurse Practitioner Faculties [NONPF], 2009).

The establishment of the DNP degree option will further broaden the range of skills to be developed by the APN, and create opportunities for additional specialty roles as the health care system changes. Mangan (2009) reports that around 80 nursing schools now offer DNP eductional programs, and the degree should allow APNs to practice more independently in a variety of clinical settings. The new doctoral degree, together with the consensus statement for regulatory reform, will bring major change to nursing, allowing nurses further independence of judgment and action.

OPPORTUNITIES FOR GROWTH

Health care reform approaches will provide opportunities for APNs to respond to the need for preventive, primary care for patients, families, and communities. The number of uninsured Americans who may be covered and then seek primary care, taken together with the shortage of primary care physicians, estimated at 30%, will mean that APNs will be in great demand (Pickert, 2009). Some health care reform plans have incorporated language that includes NPs and PAs in providing primary care. Of course, other APNs will also be called upon to provide coverage in hospitals, home health, and other agencies, as expanded coverage becomes available.

A hospital-based opportunity for APNs may result from limitations that are placed on medical resident hours. As Olson and Chioffi (2005) discuss, 80-hour/week restrictions enacted by the Accreditation Council for Graduate Medical Education in 2000 may necessitate delegation of medical tasks to other health professionals. Whether APNs will have this opportunity rests with the nursing and medical professions to resolve.

SUMMARY

The best policy options are guided by ethical insights and legal openness to change based on societal realities. Justice dictates that APNs should be able to practice their profession alongside physicians with compensation that reflects their skill, effort, and responsibilities. Patients, families, and communities benefit from the added choice of provider. The regulatory consensus statement (NCSBN, 2008) offers an opportunity to build a coordinated, consistent approach to educational, licensure, certification, and accreditation requirements nationally. APNs have been very successful in gaining acceptance within nursing and outside nursing for expanded roles and responsibilities. The public has embraced the expanded roles, but those health professionals, primarily physicians, who view the expansion of nursing as competitive and of lesser quality than their own practices, have resisted the expansion.

As APNs develop their strategies to achieve the tenets of the consensus model, their strength will be in coalitions with those individuals and groups in support of their efforts. Businesses such as retail clinics have a vested interest in the success of the APNs who work there. Hospitals need high-quality, cost-effective health providers to care for patients, and will explore and adopt APN roles that evolve in their states. Most of all, consumers will provide effective voices in support of APNs. Patients who have experienced the care provided by CNSs, NPs, CRNAs, and CNMs will step forward in legislative hearings to testify to the high-quality care they received. They will also support APN efforts to obtain whistleblowing and reimbursement legislation with the teeth to make a difference.

KEY POINTS

1. Public and private organizations both build health care policy and APNs need to work with both to make changes.
2. The consensus statement published by the National Council of State Boards of Nursing in 2008 will synchronize policy choices among states to achieve patient access and safety.
3. Political strategy that incorporates consumers will be most effective in bringing the consensus statement to fruition.
4. APNs need to know the myriad legal requirements before billing governmental or private insurers, or before choosing to report billing or reimbursement fraud.
5. Retail stores offer rich opportunities for APNs to provide care to their patients.
6. Health care reform proposals offer options for APNs to provide preventive, primary care services to patients and their communities.

REFERENCES

American Association of Colleges of Nursing (AACN). (2009, April). *Fact sheet: The doctor of nursing practice (DNP)*. Retrieved August 11, 2009, from http://www.aacn.n che.edu/Media/pdf/FS_dnp.pdf
American Association of Nurse Practitioners (AANP). (2007). *Standards for nurse practitioner practice in retail-based clinics*. Retrieved April 18, 2010, from http://www. aanp.org/NR/rdonlyres/9429B4BC-AB09-4CB6-A699-EB5AC43852D6/0/RetailBased Clinics.pdf
American Nurses Association (ANA). (2009, July). *Whistleblower protection*. Retrieved August 18, 2009, from http://www.nursingworld.org/MainMenuCategories/ ANAPoliticalPower/ State/StateLegislativeAgenda/Whistleblower_1.aspx

Anti-kickback Laws, 42 U.S.C. § 1320a-7b (1994).

Barbee, D. (2009, July 17). *Two nurses who complained about physician are indicted.* Retrieved August 17, 2009, from http://www.star-telegram.com/health/story/1493326.html

Bowring-Lossock, E. (2006). The forensic mental health nurse—A literature review. *Journal of Psychiatric and Mental Health Nursing, 13*(6), 780–785.

Buppert, C. (2005). *The primary care provider's guide to compensation and quality: How to get paid and not get sued* (2nd ed). Sudbury, MA: Jones & Bartlett.

Buppert, C. (2008). Three states auditing NPs for compliance with regulations. *Journal for Nurse Practitioners, 4*(7), 508–509.

Buppert, C. (2009). Billing issues for nurse practitioners who provide inpatient services. *Topics in Advanced Practice Nursing eJournal, 9*(1). Retrieved April 18, 2010, from http://www.medscape.com/viewarticle/705683

False Claims Act, 31 U.S.C.A. § 3729-3731 (1982).

Hannigan, N. S. (2006). Blowing the whistle on healthcare fraud: Should I? *Journal of the Amercan Academy of Nurse Practitioners, 18*(11), 512–517.

Hsu, A. (2008). Legal issues concerning retail clinics. *Health Lawyer, 20*(5), 13–28.

Inglis, T. (2009, August 3). Retaliation against West Texas nurses is unacceptable. *Austin-American Statesman,* A11.

Landro, L. (2008, April 2). Making room for 'Dr. Nurse.' *Wall Street Journal,* p. D1.

Mangan, K. (2009). A new degree and exam create 'doctor nurses,' irking physicians. *Chronicle of Higher Education.* Retrieved April 18, 2010, from http://chronicle.com/weekly/v55/i19/19a00701.htm

Mason, D. J., Leavitt, J. K., & Chaffee, M. W. (2007). *Policy & politics in nursing and health care* (5th ed.). St. Louis, MO: Saunders.

Miller, K. P. (2008). Legal liability in convenient care clinics: Much ado about nothing. *Journal for Nurse Practitioners, 4*(10), 773–775.

National Council of State Boards of Nursing (NCSBN). (2008, July). *Consensus model for APRN regulation: Licensure, accreditation, certification & education.* Retrieved April 18, 2010, from https://www.ncsbn.org/7_23_08_Consensue_APRN_Final.pdf

National Organization of Nurse Practitioner Faculties (NONPF). (2009, June). *Clarification of nurse practitioner specialty and sub-specialty clinical track titles, hours and credentialing.* Retrieved April 18, 2010, from http://www.nonpf.org/associations/10789/files/ProjectFinalReport. pdf

Olson, D. M., & Chioffi, S. M. (2005). Restrictions on medical resident hours: Advanced practice nurses as a workforce solution. *Journal of Nursing Law, 10*(2), 115–121.

Phillipsen, N. C., Setlow, P. D., & Jacob, I. S. (2008). The most costly billing practices ever. *Journal for Nurse Practitioners, 4*(10), 761–765.

Pickert, K. (2009, August 3). If a health-care bill passes, nurse practitioners could be key. *Time.* Retrieved August 4, 2009, from http://www.time.com/time/nation/article/0,8599,1914222,00.html

Pulcini, J., & Hart, M. A. (2007). Politics of advanced practice nursing. In D. J. Mason, J. K. Leavitt, & M. W. Chafee (Eds.), *Policy & politics in nursing and health care* (5th ed., p. 568). St. Louis, MO: Saunders.

Rickard, L. (2009). Helping clients increase profits through the use of non-physician practitioners. *Health Lawyer, 21*(5), 44–46.

Rozga, K. (2009). Retail health clinics: How the next innovation in market-driven health care is testing state and federal law. *American Journal of Law & Medicine, 35*(1), 205–231.

Safriet, B. (2002). Closing the gap between *can* and *may* in health-care providers' scopes of practice: A primer for policymakers. *Yale Journal on Regulation, 19*, 301–334.

Stanley, J. (2009). Reaching consensus on a regulatory model: What does this mean for APRNs? *Journal for Nurse Practitioners, 5*(2), 99–104.

Stark II, 42 U.S.C. § 1395nn (1998).

The American Association of Nurse Attorneys. (2005). *Business and legal guidebook for nurse practitioners.* Columbus, OH: Author.

World Health Organization. (1977). *The international statistical classification of diseases* (9th ed.). Geneva, Switzerland: Author.

4

Malpractice/Negligence

EDITH ANN BROUS

Built on a foundation of urban legend mixed with the occasional true story, supported by selective references to academic studies, and repeated so often that even the mythmakers forget the exaggeration, half truth, and outright misinformation employed in the service of their greater good, the medical malpractice myth has filled doctors, patients, legislators, and voters with the kind of fear that short circuits critical thinking.

—Tom Baker

INTRODUCTION

Although health care providers are socialized to believe that every patient is a potential plaintiff, the fear of civil liability far exceeds the reality. The unfortunate and mistaken belief that all patients represent legal liability creates a potential adversarial tone in provider–patient relationships, which is as unnecessary as it is counterproductive. Error reduction and safety improvements are critical concerns in clinical practice, but they cannot be effectively addressed unless the advanced practice nurse (APN) has a realistic understanding of liability exposure.

This chapter discusses the nature and elements of a malpractice claim, expert witness testimony, causes of action, and theories of liability. The cases selected as examples demonstrate the process and requirements for various complaints against or involving health care providers. The reader is advised, however, to incorporate them within a context of knowledge that it is the rare patient who files a lawsuit, pursues a claim to trial, and ultimately prevails with the jury.

APNs have ethical and professional responsibilities to advocate for their patients. The environment in which care is provided determines, in great part, whether or not the patient is protected from injury. Safety experts and regulators alike advise providers to cultivate cultures of safety in which errors are reported, analyzed, and used as opportunities to improve systems. Unfounded or exaggerated fears of litigation compromise transparency, disclosure, integrity, and honest dialogue with patients. As such, they compromise patient safety and erode the provider–patient relationship. Patients do not decide to call lawyers solely for monetary reasons. At times, the motivation is fueled by a belief that adequate information can only be obtained by instituting legal action. APNs who are perceived as honest, forthright, and accountable are less likely to be sued, because their patients are less likely to think they need an outside advocate to answer their questions.

Although tort reform proponents, politicians, and medical societies promote a great deal of misinformation regarding runaway juries, defensive medicine, multimillion dollar awards, physicians quitting medical practice because of the malpractice "crisis," "junk lawsuits," or "frivolous lawsuits," an objective look at the actual statistics reveals that the evidence basis for these claims is missing (Hunter, 2007). This chapter will discuss realistic sources of liability, common claims brought against APNs, the necessary elements in prosecuting a negligence claim, and suggestions for reducing exposure. All nurses should critically evaluate what they are told about malpractice exposure and separate political rhetoric from evidence-based information. The responsibility to function as a patient advocate does not cease when something goes wrong. Indeed, it may be at this point that such advocacy is most critical.

BACKGROUND

The vast majority of patients (approximately 98%) who have been harmed by medical negligence do not bring lawsuits (Mello, 2006a). Of those complaints that are filed, 10 times more claims are dropped than pursued (Smarr, 2005). Most medical malpractice lawsuits (almost 70%) are dismissed or settled, and do not actually proceed to trial (Schmitt, 2008). Of those that are pursued to trial, approximately 70–

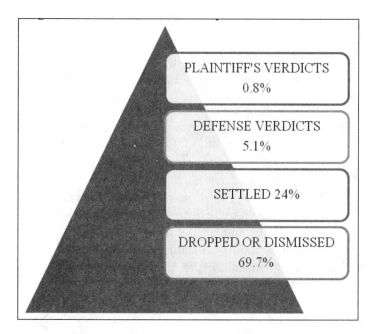

Figure 4.1 Outcome of malpractice cases closed in 2003.

Source: Physician Insurers Association of America, Testimony of Lawrence E. Smarr, President, Illinois General Assembly, House Judiciary April 7, 2005.

86% of jury decisions result in defense verdicts (General Accounting Office, 2003). Figure 4.1 illustrates these percentages.

Health care providers have been inundated with assertions that frivolous lawsuits, runaway juries, greedy lawyers, and a malpractice "crisis" are responsible for rising medical costs. Malpractice litigation, however, only accounts for 2–3% of the nation's health care bill. The public has been told that providers are leaving practice because malpractice insurance premiums have risen in response to increased litigation and high jury awards. There is no evidence that either of these claims is valid. To the contrary, multiple studies indicate that the number of malpractice lawsuits has leveled or even declined, and the supply of physician services has been affected minimally, if at all, by the malpractice environment (Mello, 2006b, North Carolina Advocates for Justice, 2009).

As Marlynn Wei has noted:

The [American Medical Association] Code of Ethics clearly forbids physicians from considering legal liability during disclosure, but fear of malpractice litigation is pervasive and potent. Physicians see the tort system as an irrational "lawsuit lottery" and "revile malpractice claims as random events that visit unwarranted expense and emotional pain on competent, hardworking practitioners." But physicians overestimate the certainty and severity of legal sanctions, and the actual risk of getting sued by threefold. Studies suggest that physicians believe erroneously that most negligent adverse events lead to lawsuits, estimating that sixty percent of cases involving negligence result in litigation, which is thirty times higher than most estimates. (Wei, 2007, pp. 137–138, footnotes omitted)

Malpractice premiums have risen in response to many economic factors. Industry price wars, stock market losses, economic cycles, declining profitability, market volatility, and investment practices of the insurance companies account for the rising prices of malpractice policies, not the litigious nature of patients, as is claimed (Boothman, Blackwell, Campbell, Commiskey, & Anderson, 2009). Premium spikes are related, in part, to the economic cycle of insurers and declines in investment income, not rising numbers of claims or "megaverdicts" (Hunter, Cassell-Stiga, & Doroshow, 2009). Indeed, the increase in malpractice premiums has not kept up with the increase in medical costs. Although medical costs have increased by 113% since 1987, the amount spent on medical malpractice insurance has increased by just 52% over that time.

Malpractice litigation *is* expensive, and premium increases may reflect those costs (Studdart, 2006). The insurance company that does defend a malpractice claim can incur great expense in doing so, regardless of the outcome. The use of the court system may not be the most cost-effective manner of resolving disputes, but is seen by injured patients as the only redress available. Efforts to address the inefficiencies and expenses of the court system would also address the issue more directly and fairly. Reducing medical error and improving provider–patient relationships is a more effective and just approach to reducing malpractice costs than imposing restrictions on the plaintiff's ability to hold negligent providers accountable. Providers interested in reducing liability should recognize that patients sue for a variety of reasons. Most patients who file legal actions are angry, frustrated, and discouraged. Perceptions that they are unable to obtain honest explanations make them feel helpless and betrayed, even bitter. They may also hope the lawsuit will prevent injury to future patients. Provider–patient relationships are pivotal in preventing these perceptions and in reducing lawsuits.

NEGLIGENCE AND MALPRACTICE

Negligence and malpractice actions occur within a body of law called *tort law*. A tort is simply a compensable civil wrong committed by one person against another. It is distinguished from a criminal act or contract violation. The injured party may hold the *tortfeasor* liable and seek compensation for the damages. Torts may be intentional or unintentional. Defamation, involuntary imprisonment, assault, battery, fraud, trespass, conversion, and the intentional infliction of emotional distress are some examples of intentional torts. Negligence, malpractice, and negligent infliction of emotional distress, on the other hand, are examples of unintentional torts (Keeton, Dobbs, Keeton, & Owen). Nursing malpractice cases are based upon the negligence theory of a duty of reasonable care.

Negligence and *malpractice* are not interchangeable terms. Although both refer to unintentional acts that cause harm to another person, there are important distinctions. The statute of limitations may be different, the need for expert witnesses differs, and the standards of proof or procedural requirements may differ as well.

Negligence is a broad term and is defined as the failure to act as a reasonably prudent person would act in same or similar circumstances. This is a lay standard and does not usually require the testimony of an expert witness. There may need to be evidence of foreseeability. The test for foreseeability is whether a person of ordinary intelligence would have anticipated the danger his or her negligence created. In other words, a reasonable person of average intelligence would be able to anticipate the consequences of the APN's negligent behavior. Foreseeability of the actual injury suffered may not be necessary to pursue the claim.

Malpractice is a specific form of professional negligence, and is defined as the failure to adhere to generally accepted standards of practice and act as a reasonably prudent professional would in same or similar circumstances. This is a standard that does require the testimony of an expert witness. Expert witnesses for both the plaintiff and the defense testify that in their opinion, to a reasonable degree of medical certainty, the defendant did or did not render care in accordance with generally accepted standards of practice. Traditionally, those standards were defined by a "locality" rule, in which the provider's conduct was compared with what other providers in the same community would do. The trend in many jurisdictions has been to abandon the locality rule and look at the defendant's actions within the context of national standards.

Tesoro v. Alvarez (2009) exemplifies the importance of distinguishing between negligence and malpractice. In this case, a family nurse practitioner (FNP) at an aesthetic clinic performed hair removal on a patient's legs using a MeDioStar HC laser. The client filed a complaint, alleging that the FNP's improper use of the laser burned her legs. Her suit also named the clinic's physician, claiming he was vicariously liable for the FNP's actions. (Vicarious liability is discussed in more detail below.)

The doctor attempted to have the complaint dismissed (by filing a *motion to dismiss*) on the basis that the client (plaintiff) had not filed an expert report as required under the state's medical liability code.[1] The plaintiff responded that the code only required expert reports for "health care liability" claims (malpractice), and laser hair removal did not involve the practice of medicine or constitute health care. Because her complaint alleged general *negligence*, not medical *malpractice*, expert reports were not required. The trial court agreed and denied the physician's motion to dismiss her complaint.

On appeal, the doctor argued that laser hair removal did constitute health care because the plaintiff referred to it as "treatment" in her complaint; the procedure took place in a medical clinic with a regulated medical device; and it involved obtaining a medical history and physical assessment, generation of a medical record, and informed consent. The appeals court stated that the plaintiff's allegations only asserted improper use of the laser; they did not assert that the FNP had deviated from acceptable standards of medical or nursing care.

The complaint was framed as a common law (determined by case law, not statute) negligence claim that the FNP negligently used the laser and that the physician was vicariously liable for her actions. The court confirmed that there may be claims arising from health care settings that are properly classified as common law negligence and not health care liability claims. Additionally, the state did not regulate laser hair removal, nor did it mandate that the procedure be performed by a health care professional. The claim, therefore, was not one of health care liability. As such, no expert report was required, and the court upheld the denial of the physician's motion to dismiss.

Similarly, in *Snyder v. Injured Patients and Families* (2009), a locked inpatient psychiatric unit failed to conduct a body or possessions search of a patient returning from a 5-hour leave. As such, the staff did not discover a handgun and ammunition in her clothing. The staff also failed to uncover the handgun and ammunition in a room search on the day of her return, or again on the following day. The patient subsequently fatally shot herself. Her husband brought suit against the facility. He sought a declaratory ruling (an opinion issued by the judge, which declares the rights of the parties) from the court that the claim was one for wrongful death, not malpractice, and was therefore not subject to the state's medical malpractice requirements.

The hospital argued that the claim was a claim related to health care services because it involved actions of hospital employees during the course of their employment. The court disagreed, holding that the conducting of a search was a ministerial and custodial function, not a medical task. (*Ministerial* or *custodial* activities are those that do not require independent decision making. They are contrasted with *discretionary* responsibilities, which do require the exercise of professional judgment.) The court concluded that the claimed failure to search the decedent alleged ordinary negligence, not medical malpractice. The case was allowed to go forward as a negligence claim, not subject to the state's medical malpractice requirements.

ELEMENTS OF A CLAIM

For a plaintiff to prevail in a medical malpractice lawsuit, he or she must prove each of the following elements: duty, breach, causation, and harm. In some states, the plaintiff may be required to submit to a presuit malpractice screening panel before pursuing a claim in a court of law. Many states that once used such panels have abandoned them, finding that they simply added another expensive layer to the litigation process or that they actually increased the number of claims (Wei, 2007, p. 156).

Duty

In the absence of a duty, there can be no liability for malpractice. In the context of a provider–patient relationship, APNs have an obligation to provide care within generally accepted standards of practice. The standards are determined by evidence-based research; expert witness testimony; internal policies and procedures; Nurse Practice Acts; local, state, and federal laws; and professional organizations. The duty is created with the establishment of a patient–provider relationship, and is generally defined as the exercise of the degree of skill ordinarily employed by an APN under similar circumstances. The duty is to use reasonable care and diligence, along with best judgment, in the application of skill to the case. Although this may ordinarily require expert testimony to establish, there are exceptions, as illustrated in *Odom v. State* (1999).

In this wrongful-death case, a 15-year-old boy died of hypoxia in a state facility. The child had been born 12 weeks prematurely, weighing 1.6 pounds, and suffering from hyaline membrane disease, spastic quadriplegia, hydrocephaly, asthma, a convulsive disorder, respiratory distress, and profound mental retardation. Additionally, a malformation of the head, neck, and trachea caused obstructive apnea, for which he depended on a tracheotomy to breathe. His written care plan included the constant use of an apnea monitor with specific parameters for the alarms. An explicit physician's order stated that the alarms were to be kept on at all times.

On nursing rounds, the child was found with the tracheotomy tube out of the stoma, but still tightly attached to his neck. His color was blue and there were no respirations or palpable pulse. A resident training specialist who was unaware that the child had a tracheotomy initiated cardiopulmonary resuscitation by ventilating through the patient's mouth. An unsuccessful attempt was made to reinsert the tracheotomy tube. There was no spare tracheotomy tube at the bedside, as was also required. The alarm never sounded.

The family motioned the court for a directed verdict and the court granted this motion, submitting the case to the jury to determine damages. (A *directed verdict* is an order from the judge directing the outcome of the case and determining who prevails in the dispute.) The jury awarded the adoptive mother $86,000 and the adoptive father $8,000 in general damages. The jury also awarded the adoptive parents $75,000 for the child's predeath fright and pain, and $3,394 in funeral and burial expenses. The trial court increased the medical expense damages from $1,215 to $1,992.34, and the state facility appealed.

The Court of Appeal of Louisiana, Third Circuit, agreed with the trial court in stating:

> [T]he degree of skill that the nurses at Pinecrest were supposed to employ, viewed in light of the degree of skill ordinarily employed under similar circumstances by the members of the nursing profession in good standing in the same community or locality, required them, simply, to follow the order issued, either by Dr. Baroni at the children's hospital or Pinecrest's own doctors regarding the operation of the apnea monitor: namely, the nurses had to leave the monitor on at all times, in the least, when Jojo was left unattended and/or while he slept....[T]he nurses still were under

the duty to place Jojo on a heart monitor while he lay in bed unattended. (*Odom v. State*, p. 97)

The trial court found that the nurses at Pinecrest failed in their duty to keep the monitor on and that reasonable minds could not reach a contrary verdict. Again, we agree. The evidence adduced at trial regarding this issue is overwhelming. It is undisputed that the nurses did not hear the monitor's alarm sound at all times pertinent to the events....testimony eliminates any other possibilities except that the monitor was turned off or that it was on but not reset after the alarm sounded at some time during the day. (*Odom v. State*, p. 98)

In *Quirk v. Zuckerman* (2003), a man presented to an emergency room complaining of right elbow pain. Swelling was noted, and he was triaged to the fast treatment area where he was examined by a nurse practitioner (NP). Noting the X-ray to be normal, the NP diagnosed epicondylitis. She placed the arm in a sling, advised the patient to ice it and keep it elevated, prescribed pain medication, and directed the patient to follow up with an orthopedist. The hospital did not have a written protocol regarding the use of NPs. The emergency department's attending physician signed the record after consulting with the NP, but did not examine the patient himself. The patient returned the following morning and was diagnosed with compartment syndrome. He developed irreversible tissue damage, necessitating amputation.

When the patient brought suit, the physician claimed that his involvement with the patient was limited to approval of the NP's diagnosis and treatment. He denied having any duty to independently examine the patient, thus refuting that a provider–patient relationship existed. To evaluate this claim, the court examined the relationship between the physician and the NP. New York state law defines NP practice as including diagnosis of illness and physical conditions, and the performance of therapeutic and corrective measures in "collaboration" with a licensed physician, although it does not define "collaboration." The Court stated that:

The nature of the relationship which constitutes collaboration is rather left to the proviso that all services be performed in accordance with a written practice agreement and written practice protocols which shall contain explicit provisions for the resolution of disputes between the nurse practitioner and the collaborating physician...However, the statute is clear that if the written agreement does not so provide, then the collaborating physician's diagnosis or treatment shall prevail if there be any conflict in diagnosis...Therefore, the ultimate responsibility for diagnosis and treatment rests with the physician if the written agreement is silent. (*Quirk v. Zuckerman*, p. 499)

The Court reasoned that the ultimate responsibility for diagnosis and treatment rested with the doctor in the absence of a written protocol by the hospital. "An implied physician–patient relationship can arise when a physician gives advice to a patient, even if the advice is communicated through another health care professional" (*Quirk v. Zuckerman*, p. 499). As such, the Court refused to dismiss the suit against the physician.

Although APNs may be permitted to render a diagnosis, the extent and nature of the collaborative practice agreement with the physician determines the potential liability for misdiagnosis on the APN's part. The APN's duty may be defined by the communication of the APN's diagnostic impressions to the physician. This is illustrated in *Siegel v. Husak* (2006). Mr. Husak injured his arms while weight-lifting and was seen by an NP in Dr. Feldman's office. The NP noted that Husak related a history of feeling immediate pain and of hearing a popping sound in his arms at the time of the injury. The NP diagnosed his arm pain as muscle strain or sprain. Contrary to the practice and protocol between the physician and the NP, Dr. Feldman did not examine or review the NP's chart to indicate agreement or disagreement with her diagnosis.

Approximately 6 months later, Mr. Husak was seen by an orthopedic surgeon, who diagnosed torn biceps tendons. The patient underwent reconstructive surgery and brought suit against Dr. Feldman and the NP. His expert witness testified that Husak would have had a greater change of full recovery had the surgery been performed within the first 10 days after the injury. The jury awarded Mr. Husak $1,848,068.50, apportioning 50% of the fault to Dr. Feldman. The Court denied the NP's motion for a judgment notwithstanding the verdict and she appealed. (A *judgment notwithstanding the verdict*, also called a *judgment as a matter of law*, is a ruling by the judge at the conclusion of a jury trial in which the judge overrules or amends the jury's decision. The motion by a party asking for this relief is rarely granted. The judge will only grant this motion when believing that the jury incorrectly applied the law, or that no reasonable jury could have arrived at the same conclusion.)

The District Court of Appeal of Florida, Third District, noted that the Florida law expressly stated that APNs could only perform diagnosis pursuant to a formal protocol between the APN and the supervising physician, and that in all circumstances, the physician "shall maintain supervision for directing the specific course of medical treatment" (*Siegel v. Husak*, p. 213). The Court held that because the NP was working under the direct supervision of Dr. Feldman, and because she did not commit any negligence apart from that for which Dr. Feldman had the ultimate responsibility, her motion should have been granted.

The APN's duty in this case was to place the information in Mr. Husak's chart so Dr. Feldman could render the correct diagnosis. The NP did chart that the patient heard a popping sound, suggestive of a ruptured tendon. Had Dr. Feldman followed the internal protocol, which required him to review the chart and agree or disagree with the NP's diagnosis, he could have diagnosed the ruptured tendon at that time. The Court held that the NP, acting under the direction of a physician, absent her own negligence, was absolved from liability for the physician's misdiagnosis. Under Florida law, the NP owed no specific duty to Husak to properly diagnose him.

Duty to Third Parties

In some cases, the provider may be held liable to third parties. *Coombes v. Florio* (2007) is an example of the concept of duty being expanded past the direct provider–patient relationship. Dr. Florio prescribed Oxycodone, Zaroxolyn, Prednisone, Flomax, potassium, Paxil, Oxazepam, and Furosemide to 75-year-old David Sacca. When Mr. Sacca was being treated for cancer, Dr. Florio warned him not to drive. When the treatment was concluded, Dr. Florio advised him that he could safely resume driving. Mr. Sacca subsequently drove his car and lost consciousness while behind the wheel. The car veered onto the sidewalk, striking and killing 10-year-old Kevin Coombs.

Kevin's estate sued Dr. Florio, claiming that he failed to warn Mr. Sacca about the side effects of the medications he was taking and that it would be dangerous for him to drive. The trial court dismissed the case, holding that Dr. Florio did not owe a duty of care to anyone but his patients. In the absence of a physician–patient relationship between the plaintiff and the defendant, the essential element of duty was not present to allow a malpractice claim.

On appeal, the Supreme Judicial Court of Massachusetts stated that the risk of harm to another person was foreseeable, and that Dr. Florio's duty of reasonable care included warning him about the side effects of medications he was prescribing. The side effects of the particular medications prescribed for Mr. Sacca included drowsiness, fainting, dizziness, and the potential for diminished mental capacity.

> In the case of automobile accidents, it is clear that the foreseeable risk of injury is not limited to the patient ....When a doctor prescribes medication

it is both a foreseeable and intended result that a patient will take the medication. The occurrence of known side effects, and the impact of such side effects on the patient's ability to drive, are foreseeable results of that prescription ....Any duty that Dr. Florio owed to warn of the side effects of medication he prescribed extended not only to Sacca, but to those whose injuries were foreseeably caused by the resulting accident....It was Dr. Florio's own act of prescribing medication that created the foreseeable risk of an accident, and his duty to warn flows from that act and extends to all those foreseeably put at risk by it. (*Coombes v. Florio*, pp. 188–194)

[W]hen a physician who has knowledge of a danger that may be posed to others from a patient's decision to operate a motor vehicle while under the influence of prescribed medication (a danger of which the public has no way of knowing) does not warn the patient of the risks involved, the physician may be held liable for injuries to others caused by the failure to warn. (*Coombes v. Florio*, p. 196)

The Court held that a physician is required to warn patients that prescribed medications have potentially dangerous side effects, such as drowsiness or loss of consciousness. Because Dr. Florio was in a position of authority in the physician–patient relationship, he was required to attempt to influence Mr. Sacca's behavior on matters within the scope of that relationship. He could have avoided the risk to Kevin by warning Mr. Sacca not to drive. The lower court's dismissal of the case was overturned, and the family was allowed to proceed against Dr. Florio.

Psychiatric nurse practitioners treating dangerous patients should be aware that some jurisdictions also expand the duty element to third parties. In *Tarasoff v. Regents of University of California* (1996), a paranoid schizophrenic patient, Prosenjit Poddar, identified to psychologist Dr. Lawrence Moore that he intended to kill Tatiana Tarasoff. Dr. Moore had Mr. Poddar detained by the police, but they released him when he appeared rational. Dr. Moore's supervisor then directed that no further action be taken to admit him. Mr. Poddar subsequently stabbed Tatiana Tarasoff to death.

Tatiana's parents brought suit, alleging that the defendants were liable for her death because it proximately resulted from their failure to warn Tatiana or others likely to tell her of the danger. The defendants argued that they had no duty to Tatiana. The Supreme Court of California held that the therapists could not escape liability merely because Tatiana herself was not the patient: "[W]hen a therapist determines, or pursuant to the standards of his profession should determine, that his patient presents a serious danger of violence to another, he incurs an obligation to use reasonable care to protect the intended victim against such danger" (*Tarasoff v. Regents of University of California*, p. 431).

The Court held that the relationship between a psychotherapist and a patient constitutes a "special relationship" that supports affirmative duties to third parties. The therapist has a duty not only to the patient himself, but also to other persons the therapist knows to be threatened by the patient. The Court also addressed concerns of therapist–patient privilege in stating that, "[t]he protective privilege ends where the public peril begins" (*Tarasoff v. Regents of University of California*, p. 442). There is no breach of professional ethics in such disclosure, as the public policy of averting danger to others outweighs the privilege of confidentiality. Such warnings are frequently referred to as *Tarasoff* warnings.

Many jurisdictions interpret *Tarasoff* narrowly in recognition of the provider's duty to protect patient confidentiality. In *People v. Bierenbaum* (2002), a plastic surgeon appealed his conviction for second-degree murder in the death of his wife. He argued, among other things, that the trial court should not have permitted evidence regarding communications between mental health professionals and his wife. Dr. Bierenbaum had seen a psychologist and two psychiatrists, and had given permission for each of them to speak with his wife. Each of them became concerned that he would harm his wife. The psychologist called her to ensure her safety and the two psychiatrists gave her *Tarasoff* warnings, one of which was in writing. The trial court did not permit the prosecution to examine the mental health providers, holding that doing so would breach provider–patient privilege. The court did allow the prosecution to introduce evidence about the *Tarasoff* warnings, however.

On appeal, the prosecution argued that the therapist–patient privilege had been waived when Dr. Bierenbaum gave the providers his permission to speak with his wife. It further argued that the *Tarasoff* warnings themselves constituted such a breach. Dr. Bierenbaum argued that the introduction of information about the *Tarasoff* warnings constituted a breach of the provider–patient privilege. The Appellate Division agreed with the trial court, which had stated that the privilege was not absolute: "[n]otwithstanding this duty to maintain confidentiality, where a patient is a danger to himself or to others, a mental health professional may be required to disclose otherwise confidential information to the extent necessary to protect a threatened interest" (*People v. Robert Bierenbaum*, 2002). The *Tarasoff* warnings in this case constituted an allowable breach for the limited purposes of protecting a potential victim of violence, and did not abrogate the provider–patient privilege. Allowing the providers to testify, however, would breach the provider–patient privilege and was not permitted.

The Appellate Division reinforced the provider's duty to potential victims, and stated that this duty could be satisfied in many ways, such as hospitalizing the patient for inpatient treatment, increasing the frequency of outpatient encounters, or the use of psychopharmacological agents. At times, the provider may have an affirmative obligation to take action in preventing potential danger. The Court stated that, "[F]or compelling policy reasons the privilege can be overcome when the patient demonstrates that he poses a clear and present danger to a third party" (*People v. Bierenbaum*, 2002, p. 142).

Breach

An APN breaches his or her duty to a patient when departing from acceptable standards of practice. Expert witnesses for both the plaintiff and the defense review the medical record, and formulate an opinion as to whether or not the APN's conduct was in accordance with the standard of practice at the time of the event. For this reason, it is important to keep old policies when they are revised. The APN needs to demonstrate compliance with the policies that were in place at the time of the alleged malpractice.

In *Hypolite v. Columbia Dauterive Hospital* (2007), a plaintiff claimed that negligent medical and nursing care led to her ruptured uterus and subsequent hysterectomy. Labor was induced with the administration of Cytotec. The patient became hypertensive and fetal bradycardia was observed. A cesarean section was performed, and after removal of the placenta and membranes, a tear was discovered in the uterus. Additionally, a broad ligament hematoma dissected into the upper part of the uterus and lateral wall, leaving only a 3–4-centimeter connection of the uterus to the cervix. Because the damage was severe and the patient was bleeding heavily, a total abdominal hysterectomy was performed.

The plaintiff alleged that the nurse midwives breached the standard of care required under the circumstances in that they: (a) failed to properly monitor and timely respond to her distress following insertion of the Cytotec pills, (b) failed to obtain her informed consent for the use of Cytotec to induce labor, (c) failed to timely summon a doctor when expert medical attention was needed, and (d) acted unreasonably by administering Cytotec to her without a specific physician's order directing its use.

At trial, both sides presented experts as to the standards of care. The plaintiff's expert witness testified that a cervical examination was necessary prior to using Cytotec, and the midwives breached the standard of care in not performing such an examination. The nursing documentation, however, refuted this claim, as the prenatal flow sheet reflected that a cervical examination had been performed prior to the decision to induce. The contention that the plaintiff was not informed of the risks and benefits of Cytotec was similarly refuted. Testimony was offered that the nurse midwife counseled the plaintiff regarding the risks and benefits of Cytotec, as well as the pros and cons of labor versus cesarean delivery, and that this conversation was witnessed by a nurse.

The plaintiff claimed the midwives breached the standards of care by administering an incorrect dosage of Cytotec and without an approved order. The defense provided evidence, however, that the institution's standard protocol had been followed. The nursing documentation also refuted the plaintiff's claim that she was inadequately monitored and that a physician was not timely summoned. The nurse's notes and fetal heart rate monitoring strips demonstrated that there was no breach in the standard of practice for observing and reporting. The Court held that:

> [A] uterine tear was a possible complication that accompanies a course of labor and that the occurrence here did not absolutely signify a breach of the physician's or nursing staffs' standard of care....Ms. Hypolite failed to establish breaches of the standards of care. (*Hypolite v. Columbia Dauterive Hospital*, p. 247)

Causation

Even when successfully demonstrating that the APN departed from acceptable standards of practice, the plaintiff will not prevail unless he or she can also demonstrate that the departure caused the injury. Different jurisdictions define causation differently, but there are common standards used to demonstrate that the harm resulted from the APN's breach of duty. Common terms include *actual cause, cause in fact, but for, proximate cause, superseding* or *intervening cause*, and *loss of chance or lost chance*.

Actual cause, also called *cause in fact*, is a *but for* standard, meaning the injury would not have occurred *but for* the provider's departure from standards. *Proximate cause* is a legal finding that the defendant's actions were the cause of the plaintiff's injury. A *superseding* or *intervening* cause is the unforeseen and independent action of another party or event that causes harm. It may reduce or eliminate liability for the original tortfeasor, but it must be unforeseen to do so. An example of the need for unforeseeability of the intervening cause is provided in *Pruette v. Phoebe Putney Memorial Hospital* (2008).

In this wrongful-death lawsuit, a patient was resuscitated from a respiratory arrest under the direction of a pulmonary critical care physician, Dr. Ungarino. She began breathing independently, but with labored respirations. The patient's private physician intervened to prevent intubation, stating the patient did not wish to be resuscitated. He subsequently ordered that 2 milligrams of morphine be administered every 30 minutes to 1 hour as needed for comfort. Dr. Ungarino then ordered that she be given a single 20-milligram dose of morphine by rapid intravenous infusion.

The patient had regained consciousness when a registered nurse (RN) administered the 20-mg dose. Her eyes closed immediately, and she never regained consciousness. When she stopped breathing a few hours later, the nurses did not intervene, as they believed she did not want to be resuscitated. The patient's daughter brought suit against Dr. Ungarino and the hospital. In his defense, Dr. Ungarino claimed that the morphine he ordered was not the proximate cause of death. Instead, he contended that the decision not to resuscitate her was an intervening factor. The Court reasoned, however:

> There can be no proximate cause where there has intervened between the act of the defendant and the injury to the plaintiff, an independent, intervening, act or omission of someone other than the defendant, which was not *foreseeable* by defendant, was not triggered by defendant's act, and which was sufficient of itself to cause the injury. (*Pruette v. Phoebe Putney Memorial Hospital*, p. 14, emphasis added)

> Here, there is evidence in the record that at the time Dr. Ungarino wrote the order for the rapid infusion of 20 milligrams of morphine, he was aware that plaintiff had made a decision that Ms. Vinson should have a "Do Not Resuscitate" status and that no additional life-saving measures should be administered if she again went into respiratory arrest. Under these circumstances, even if plaintiff's decision could be construed as an intervening cause, a jury would be entitled to conclude that the decision was reasonably *foreseeable* and should have been factored into Dr. Ungarino's decision making concerning the dosage of morphine. (*Pruette v. Phoebe Putney Memorial Hospital*, p. 15, emphasis added)

Similarly, in *Pope v. Cumberland County Hospital System* (2005), multiple attempts were made to insert a fetal scalp electrode. Upon the third attempt, the fetal heart rate dropped and the provider's glove indicated bleeding. An emergency cesarean delivery was performed. The infant was born without a pulse and was resuscitated by a team of neonatal nurse practitioners (NNPs). The labor-and-delivery nurses had not communicated to the NNPs that there had been significant bleeding. The infant was subsequently transfused, but sustained irreversible brain damage as a result of the fetal bleeding.

When the family brought suit against the hospital and the physicians, the hospital argued that the failure of the NNPs to immediately transfuse the infant was an intervening cause of her injuries. The Court agreed with the hospital, and directed a verdict in favor of the labor-and-delivery nurses. On appeal, the plaintiffs presented evidence that the failure of the NNPs to immediately transfuse the infant was a *foreseeable* result of the failure of the labor-and-delivery nurses to report to the NNPs that the fetal bradycardia was associated with bleeding. The North Carolina Court of Appeals agreed with the plaintiffs, and held that the actions of the NNPs were not independent forces, which superseded the negligence of the labor-and-delivery nurses. As such, it reversed the directed verdict in favor of the hospital, and allowed the suit to proceed against the labor-and-delivery nurses.

Substantial factor means there is a reasonable degree of medical certainty that the departure was responsible for the injury. Even if other factors played a part, the particular departure alleged played a significant role in harming the patient. Without the negligence, the injury would not have occurred. This is illustrated in *Leha v. Yonkers General Hospital* (2005).

An 8-year-old girl was admitted to the hospital for the treatment of strep throat. For several months after her discharge, she continued to complain about a sore throat and was seen in the emergency room by NPs on two different occasions. In both encounters, the NPs diagnosed viral pharyngitis and an upper respiratory infection. She was also seen by a physician for an encounter related to difficulty in breathing. The emergency room physician discharged the child, but she continued to worsen. She returned the following day in congestive heart failure, for which she ultimately underwent an aortic valve replacement.

The plaintiffs alleged that the emergency department physician had been negligent in failing to diagnose the congestive heart failure. They also claimed that the damage to the child's aortic valve had been caused by undiagnosed and untreated rheumatic fever, which, in turn, was caused by undiagnosed and untreated strep throat. They alleged that the NPs had been negligent in failing to test for strep throat. The defense expert testified that the congestive heart failure was the result of an undetected congenital heart disorder. The jury found that the NPs had been negligent in failing to test the child for strep throat, but that this negligence was not a *substantial factor* in causing her injuries.

Loss of chance or lost chance is a theory in which the injured plaintiff claims the APN's negligence was the cause of a lost chance to avoid the injury. The allegation is that the APN's failure to properly diagnose, to transfer to a hospital or intervene for an emergency condition, or to seek consultation with a physician, reduced the patient's statistical opportunity to survive or avoid disability. He was, therefore, deprived of the chance to recover or avoid injury. This principle is illustrated in *Jones v. Mercy Health Center, Inc.* (2006).

A 20-year-old man presented to the emergency department with complaints of abdominal pain and constipation, accompanied by tachycardia and an elevated white blood cell count. A large amount of stool was found in his colon on X-ray. The NP diagnosed the patient with fecal impaction, and ordered an enema. Approximately 5 hours after arrival, the patient left the hospital with a prescription for stool softeners.

Within an hour, he re-presented to another emergency department in critical condition from toxic megacolon. His abdomen was grossly distended, tympanitic, and very tender. Respirations were shallow, oxygen saturation was low, and he was hypotensive and mottled. Although the presence of a surgical emergency was immediately recognized and he was rushed to the operating room to relieve the pressure on his colon, he died during surgery. The autopsy report listed the cause of death as "constipation secondary to intestinal obstruction, with megacolon, megarectum, and fecal impaction."

The trial court granted the defense motion to dismiss the mother's malpractice lawsuit on the basis that her expert witnesses did not directly state that the actions of the first emergency department *caused* his death. On appeal, the Court stated that the "loss of chance" doctrine applied when a health care provider deprived a patient of a significant chance for recovery by negligently failing to provide medical treatment. The Court held that the mother could satisfy her causation burden by showing that the first hospital's actions resulted in a substantial decrease in the chance of survival, "conditions like [the decedent's]…when he walked into Mercy Health Care that afternoon generally resulted in death 20 to 25% of the time, but…the enema reduced his chances of survival to less than 5%" (*Jones v. Mercy Health Center, Inc.*, p. 14).

Exceptions

No Fault. Some states have no-fault compensation systems for qualifying injuries. These plans are determined by statutory schemes, and may be the exclusive remedy for plaintiffs. In such jurisdictions, the plaintiff may be prohibited from pursuing a civil action or prevented from doing so until a panel makes its own determinations. Birth, vaccine, or anesthesia-related injuries are the types of events that may be covered in these plans.

Res Ipsa Loquitur. A legal doctrine called *res ipsa loquitur*[2] may be available to plaintiffs in certain cases. Translated from the Latin, *res ipsa loquitur* means, "the thing itself speaks" or "the thing speaks for itself." The evidentiary burden of duty, breach, causation, and harm are somewhat modified when this doctrine is permitted. In such cases, circumstantial evidence may allow the jury to infer negligence. Some jurisdictions require the plaintiff to show that negligence is the only possible inference under the circumstances, or that the facts and circumstances of the case would lead a reasonable person to infer negligence.

The jury is allowed to use its own common experience and knowledge to evaluate negligence and causation. The burden then may shift to the defendant to prove that the injury was not the result of negligence. Some jurisdictions still require expert testimony as to departure and causation, although others do not. Although the plaintiff has the burden of proof in a medical malpractice case, evidence that is available to the defendant may be inaccessible to the plaintiff. A *res ipsa loquitur* claim may be permitted, therefore, in the interests of justice for the injured party.

Res ipsa loquitur is generally limited to cases in which there is no direct proof of the cause of injury, and the nature of the alleged malpractice and injuries is within the common knowledge of laypersons. The plaintiff must demonstrate that the instrumentality of harm was under the defendant's (sometimes exclusive) control; the injury that occurred is of the type that does not normally occur in the absence of negligence; and the injury was not caused by the plaintiff himself, some other cause, or a third party. Such cases generally involve surgical claims related to retained foreign objects, wrong site surgery, mechanical instrument misuse, burns sustained in fires or explosions, or nerve injuries from improper positioning.

In *Kambat v. St. Francis Hospital* (1997), a patient underwent a hysterectomy. Three months postoperatively, an abdominal X-ray was obtained when she complained of stomach pain. The X-ray revealed the presence of a foreign object, and she underwent surgery again. An 18-by-18-inch laparotomy pad was discovered in her bowel and removed. She continued to deteriorate, and subsequently died a few weeks later from the infected abscess.

The family brought suit and the trial court refused to allow use of the *res ipsa loquitur* doctrine. During the trial, the defendants had argued an alternate theory of the case, in which they proposed that the sponge had not been left inside the patient, but that she had swallowed it. The jury returned a defense verdict. The family appealed to the Appellate Division, which upheld the trial court's ruling. The family continued its appeal to the New York Court of Appeals, arguing that the court had erred in not allowing the jury to consider negligence using the *res ipsa loquitur* doctrine.

The Court of Appeals overturned the Appellate Division and granted the family a new trial:

> Turning to these remaining *res ipsa loquitur* conditions, plaintiffs' evidence that similar pads were used during decedent's surgery, that decedent was unconscious throughout the operation, that laparotomy pads are not accessible to patients and that it would be anatomically impossible to swallow such pads sufficed to allow the jury to conclude that defendants had exclusive control of the laparotomy pad "at the time of the alleged act of negligence…and that it did not result from any voluntary action by the patient." (*Kambat v. St. Francis Hospital*, p. 497)

Unlike *Kambat*, *res ipsa loquitur* was not allowed in *Bibb v. Center for Pain of Montgomery* (2009). In this case, the plaintiff underwent a cervical epidural steroid injection (CESI) for neck pain. She subsequently brought a complaint against the pain center, alleging that she had lost the use of her left hand as a consequence of the anesthesiologist's negligence. The plaintiff did not offer any expert testimony, claiming that:

> [I]t was "apparent" that the loss of the use of her left hand is "in an area remote from where [she] was being treated." She averred that "[t]his type of injury does not occur in the absence of someone's negligence and the injury occurred while [Dr. Katz] was in the exclusive control of [her]

person while undergoing an injection for neck pain." (*Bibb v. Center for Pain of Montgomery*, p. 2)

Bibb contends that the doctrine of *res ipsa loquitur* applies in her case because, she says, the loss of the use of her left hand is allegedly "in no way connected to" the treatment of her neck pain. Therefore, she asserts, it requires no special knowledge to conclude that Dr. Katz was negligent in administering the CESI. (*Bibb v. Center for Pain of Montgomery*, p. 5)

The trial court granted the defendant's motion to dismiss the case and the plaintiff appealed. The Alabama Supreme Court upheld the trial court's dismissal of the case, stating that, "[I]t is indeed conceivable that a person could lose feeling in an extremity as a result of an injection near the spinal cord" (*Bibb v. Center for Pain of Montgomery*, p. 5). The Court cited a previous case, in which it was held that:

The need for expert testimony "is dependent upon whether the average person is able to decide without expert testimony whether or not the procedure followed in any given case falls below the acceptable standard....The standard of care for administering a CESI and the risks, if any, associated with administering a CESI in accordance with that standard of care are not subjects within the knowledge of the average person. The administration of the CESI involves "specialized training and knowledge that puts an understanding of the acceptable standard of care...beyond the common knowledge of the jury. Laymen do not have the background and knowledge without expert testimony to understand whether or not [the CESI] has been properly [administered]." (*Bibb v. Center for Pain of Montgomery*, p. 6)

Common Knowledge Doctrine. A rare exception to the need for expert testimony in evidencing duty, breach, causation, and harm is the common knowledge doctrine or common experience doctrine. Although related to the doctrine of *res ipsa loquitur*, there are distinctions. The plaintiff in a *res ipsa* case must prove his injury, but does not need to prove a standard of care or a specific departure from it. With the common knowledge doctrine, the plaintiff must not only prove his injury, but also some act or omission that caused that injury. Expert testimony is not necessary, because, as in a simple negligence case, the jury can provide the applicable standard of care from its common knowledge. As in *res ipsa loquitur*, the issue of negligence is not one that requires the technical expertise of a professional, but lies within the knowledge of a layperson with average intelligence and ordinary experiences.

The doctrine of common experience is illustrated in *Sanzari v. Rosenfeld* (1961). In this wrongful-death case, a dentist injected Mrs. Sanzari's gums with xylocaine containing epinephrine before replacing a filling. After the procedure, Mrs. Sanzari fell, suffered a cerebral hemorrhage, and died 3 days later. At trial, there was testimony that the epinephrine had aggravated her pre-existing hypertension, causing the cerebral hemorrhage and subsequent death. There was also testimony that the dentist was unaware of her hypertension, and that he failed to obtain a medical history prior to injecting her with the medication.

The dentist sought to have the case dismissed, in part, on the basis that there was no expert testimony regarding the standards of practice for dentists administering anesthesia. When the court did dismiss the case, the plaintiff appealed, arguing that, among other things, it had been unnecessary to establish the standard of care in this case. The Supreme Court of New Jersey overturned the dismissal and remanded it (sent it back to the trial court) for trial:

> [T]he jury could reasonably conclude that defendant knew or should have known that it was dangerous to administer epinephrine to a hypertensive patient. We believe that it is within the common knowledge of laymen that a reasonable man, including a dentist, who knows a drug is potentially harmful to a certain type of patient should take adequate precaution before administering the drug or deciding whether to administer it. The jury could reasonably conclude from the evidence that defendant took no precautions or inadequate precautions before injecting xylocaine with epinephrine into Mrs. Sanzari. (*Sanzari v. Rosenfeld*, p. 143)

The doctrine of common experience is rarely applied in medical malpractice cases, as a Hawaii case illustrates. In *Barbee v. Queens* (2008), Mr. Barbee underwent a laparoscopic nephrectomy. He was returned to surgery for internal bleeding and subsequently died 18 months later. A jury returned a plaintiffs' verdict against the hospital and surgeon. Both appealed, and their motions for judgments as a matter of law were granted. (A "renewed motion for motion for judgment as a matter of law," as it is referred to in Federal Court, is a motion in which one party asks the Court to "direct a verdict" in its favor. The party making this motion claims that the opponent's case is not supported by the evidence. If the Court finds that a reasonable jury could find for the opponent, it will deny the motion and the case will continue. If the Court finds that a reasonable jury could not find in favor of the opponent, it will grant this motion, effectively ending the case.)

In addition to granting the defendants' motions for judgment as a matter of law, the Circuit Court granted the surgeon's motion for a new trial. The family appealed, arguing that, "either there was sufficient evidence regarding the cause of death to go to the jury, or that this case falls in the exception in which expert testimony is not necessary because the cause of death is one that is within the common understanding and perception of a member of the general public" (*Barbee v. Queens*, p. 145).

The Intermediate Court of Appeals of Hawaii noted that there had been no expert testimony regarding the cause of Mr. Barbee's death and that the death occurred 18 months after the procedure:

> [I]n any event, the court does not believe that the record supports the conclusion that this is a case in which lay persons are competent to testify and offer opinions regarding cause of death...., the court is unable to find any evidence by a competent expert regarding cause of death of Mr. Lloyd Barbee. (*Barbee v. Queens*, p. 145)

Citing previous cases, the Court noted:

> Hawai'i does recognize a "common knowledge" exception to the requirement that a plaintiff must introduce expert medical testimony on causation. ...The exception is similar to the doctrine of *res ipsa loquitur*, and when applied, transforms a medical malpractice case "into an ordinary negligence case, thus obviating the necessity of expert testimony to establish the applicable standard of care."...This exception is "rare in application," ...and applies in instances such as "[w]hen an operation leaves a sponge in the patient's interior, or removes or injures an inappropriate part of his anatomy, or when a tooth is dropped down his windpipe or he suffers a serious burn from a hot water bottle, or when instruments are not sterilized[.]" (*Barbee v. Queens*, p. 159)

The plaintiffs argued that expert testimony was not required because lay persons could understand that blood loss may cause organ failure and death. The cause of Mr. Barbee's death was not so technical that it required an expert opinion to explain. Lay persons could draw their own conclusions. The Court disagreed, and held that the cause of death was not within the realm of common knowledge. In this case, the death occurred 17 months after the alleged negligence. Lay persons would need expert testimony to understand the role that the long-term effects of internal bleeding and preexisting conditions played in the death.

Understanding of such a "sophisticated injury" would not be within the realm of a reasonable jury.

Ministerial Functions. Another exception to the need for expert witness testimony exists when the negligence complained of is of a ministerial, administrative, or routine nature. In such cases, the standard of care does not require proof by an expert witness, but also falls within the realm of a lay juror's comprehension. This is illustrated in *Kujawski v. Arbor View Center* (1987). In this case, an 81-year-old nursing home patient, Angela Cieler, fell out of her wheelchair while being transported. The complaint alleged that the nursing home was negligent in "(1) not securely tying or strapping Cieler into the wheelchair; (2) pushing the wheelchair at a speed which was too fast under the conditions; (3) striking the table with the wheelchair as it was being pushed; and (4) stopping the wheelchair so abruptly as to cause the plaintiff to be thrown forward out of the chair" (*Kujawski v. Arbor View Center*, p. 458).

The trial court granted the defendant's motion to dismiss the case on the basis that no expert witness testimony had been presented regarding the standard of care the nursing home owed to the patient. The trial court reasoned that, "[A] determination of whether to use a safety belt of the type suggested by the plaintiff is not a matter within the realm of the ordinary experiences of mankind." (*Kujawski v. Arbor View Center*, p. 462). As such, expert testimony was required to establish the standard of care required by the nursing home.

This dismissal was upheld on appeal, and the plaintiff appealed to the Wisconsin Supreme Court. Arbor View argued that the use of restraints was a "medical decision" because it required a physician's order. The Supreme Court disagreed with the defendant, reversed the lower court dismissal of the suit, and sent the matter back for trial, stating:

[A] nursing home's use or non-use of a restraint involves a matter of routine care which does not need to be established through expert testimony. In this case, the decision regarding the use of a restraint under the circumstances does not involve a situation so complex or technical that a jury would need expert testimony to determine the appropriate standard of care. One does not need to be an expert to determine whether a patient who has fallen out of her wheelchair, and who is too large to fit comfortably in her wheelchair, should be secured in her wheelchair even if she has a ventral hernia. Accordingly,...expert testimony is unnecessary in this case. (*Kujawski v. Arbor View Center*, p. 464)

Arbor View's use or non-use of restraints involves a matter of routine care,…expert testimony was not required to establish the standard of care applicable to Arbor View. The decision to leave Cieler unrestrained does not involve a matter of therapy and, therefore, does not constitute a medical decision requiring expert testimony. (*Kujawski v. Arbor View Center*, p. 468)

Harm

The purpose of a lawsuit is not to create a windfall, but to make the injured party whole, or compensate the injured party for the harm. Physical, emotional, and financial harm result from malpractice. Loss of earnings, continuing medical expenses, loss of parental guidance, loss of spousal support or marital relations, funeral and burial expenses, emotional distress, pain and suffering, losses of lifestyle, and loss of life itself, are all compensable injuries. In a medical malpractice lawsuit, the plaintiff must demonstrate that the injury complained of was a direct result of the negligence.

If the plaintiff has successfully demonstrated that the defendant breached his or her duty and that the breach caused an injury, the damages to which he or she is entitled will be determined by the finder of fact. (The *finder of fact* determines issues of *fact*, not of *law*, and is a jury in a jury trial or a judge in a bench trial. This is in contrast to a *trier of law*, who determines issues of statutory construction, evidence admissibility, or other issues of *law* and is always the judge or the court.) In damage determinations, the individual circumstances of the specific case are considered to assess the particular effects of the particular injuries on the particular plaintiff.

The defendant (or defendants) responsible for the plaintiff's injury "takes the victim as he finds him," meaning the award is not based upon what an average plaintiff would need to be made whole, but what this particular plaintiff needs considering his particular vulnerabilities. The defendant will be held responsible for the consequences of his negligence, even if the consequences exceed what would ordinarily be found. The defendant may not have caused an underlying condition, but is responsible for aggravation of the plaintiff's injuries. This is sometimes referred to as the "eggshell plaintiff" or "eggshell skull" theory.

In *Brandner v. Hudson* (2007), a physician was sued for negligence and assault by a coworker. The plaintiff sought compensatory and punitive damages for a knee injury and emotional distress. Although her injuries were considered unusual, the court noted the eggshell plaintiff rule and concluded that the physician "takes his plaintiff as he finds her." It held that whether her reaction was unusual or not was irrelevant and awarded her $90,828 in compensatory damages and $25,000 in punitive damages.

The physician appealed, and the Supreme Court of Alaska affirmed the trial court's decision. Citing previous case law, the court stated, "[T]he defendant must take the victim as the defendant finds the victim and is liable for those injuries caused or aggravated by defendant's negligence....While the extent of Hudson's injury may have been unusual or unpredictable, Dr. Brandner is nonetheless liable for all injuries that were either caused or aggravated by his actions" (*Brandner v. Hudson*, p.88).

In *Wolbers v. Finley Hospital* (2003), a postoperative carotid endarterectomy patient complained about difficulty breathing. A physician attempted to intubate him but was unsuccessful, due to airway blockage. The surgeon was not notified of the problem and the patient subsequently died. In the wrongful death lawsuit, the hospital argued that the airway blockage was caused by the patient's smoking history. The court instructed the jury on the eggshell plaintiff rule as follows:

> If the decedent, Samuel Wolbers, had a condition which made him more susceptible to injury than a person in normal health, then the Defendant is responsible for all injuries and damages which are experienced by the decedent proximately caused by Defendant's...actions, even though the injuries claimed produce a greater injury than those which might have been experienced by a normal person under the same circumstances. (*Wolbers v. Finley Hospital*, pp. 736–737)

The jury returned a verdict in favor of the plaintiff and the hospital appealed, arguing that the court should have instructed the jury that the patient contributed to his own death by smoking. The Supreme Court of Iowa upheld the trial court, stating:

> While it seems clear that smoking can produce increased secretions, such as the ones that caused a blockage to the airways of plaintiff's decedent, it seems equally clear that the present claim was based on the hospital staff's alleged failure to adequately treat the condition that existed, whatever its cause. (*Wolbers v. Finley Hospital*, p. 733)

The amount of damages to which a plaintiff is entitled is established by evidence. The award is determined by what is necessary to compensate the plaintiff for the injuries. Expert testimony may be required to establish the amount, which is based upon the specific circumstances of the individual case. The trial judge has a great deal of discretion in determining that an amount is excessive, or that it was based upon "passion and prejudice." The court may also determine that the jury verdict or decision is against the weight of the evidence or is in violation of law.

Most "reform" measures are based upon the belief that attorneys and the legal system create a malpractice crisis. As such, damage awards are frequently the targets of such reform efforts. Damage caps have been imposed in many jurisdictions with the intent of making medical malpractice litigation less appealing to patients and their attorneys. Limiting potential recoveries, however, does not reduce the actual cost of litigation, nor does it deter suits from patients who feel they have been injured by negligent providers. There is no evidence that these measures reduce the number of lawsuits filed, or that they reduce their costs.

Expert Testimony

Expert testimony is generally required in medical malpractice cases because lay persons are considered to lack the knowledge required for understanding nursing practice and medical causation. Experts are used to explain the standards of practice, how the defendants deviated from those standards, and how that deviation created the injuries alleged in the complaint. The expertise of a licensed professional is generally required in establishing the plaintiff's claim, as well as in defending against it. The court determines the admissibility of expert witness testimony based upon statutory requirements, the reliability of the witness, the relevance of the witness's testimony, and the usefulness of the testimony for the jury.

The test as to whether an individual witness is competent to testify in a particular malpractice action is defined by specific statutes and interpreted differently by different jurisdictions. Generally, however, considerations include the knowledge and experience of the proposed witness, expertise in the professional standards applicable to the case, licensure in the profession, whether or not the subject matter of the situation falls within the realm of the witnesses' particular profession, and familiarity with the particular facts of the situation at issue. A member of one profession may provide expert witness testimony regarding the standards of another profession in situations in which the subject matter of the practice standards at issue falls within the province of both professions, or when there is mutual or overlapping competence.

An example of this is *Baylor Medical v. Wallace* (2009). Mr. Wallace was treated and released from the emergency department. A complaint filed by the family claimed the hospital failed to properly evaluate, diagnose, and treat him for a cerebral bleed, from which he subsequently sustained severe and permanent brain damage. The hospital filed a motion to dismiss the suit on the basis that the family had not filed an adequate expert report. The trial court denied the motion, and the hospital appealed. On appeal, the hospital argued that the plaintiff's physician expert witness was qualified to testify regarding the standards of practice for an emergency physician, but not necessarily qualified to testify regarding the standards of practice for the other health care providers in the emergency room.

The plaintiffs argued that physicians were not disqualified from offering opinions regarding nursing care, particularly because the expert report expressly referenced his experience in working with nurses, NPs, and physician's assistants, as well as his familiarity with the standards of care applicable to those providers. The Court of Appeals of Texas, Fifth District, agreed with the plaintiffs, stating:

> [I]f the physician states he is familiar with the standard of care for both nurses and physicians, and for the prevention and treatment of the illness, injury, or condition involved in the claim, the physician is qualified on the issue of whether the health care provider departed from the accepted standards of care for health care providers. (*Baylor Medical v. Wallace*, p. 558)

Similarly, in *Grover v. Isom* (2002), a dental patient had been experiencing severe right-sided headaches, which she attributed to tooth problems. In the oral surgeon's office, the certified registered nurse anesthetist (CRNA) administered Brevital while the patient underwent extraction. She did not awaken from the anesthesia as expected, and began exhibiting signs of neurological distress. The patient was transferred to a hospital, where it was determined that she had suffered a stroke. She subsequently lost the use of her left arm, had difficulty walking, and needed assistance in her daily living. At trial, the jury found that the patient's stroke had begun prior to her office visit, and that she was 100% responsible for her own injuries. The plaintiff appealed, arguing that the defense expert witness, a CRNA, had been unqualified to offer expert testimony because he had not administered anesthesia in an office setting.

The Court noted that the defense expert was licensed as a CRNA in three states and had practiced for nearly 20 years. Although he had not administered anesthesia in an office settling, he had administered anesthesia with dentists before. Additionally, the setting in which anesthesia is administered does not affect the standard of care. As such, he was qualified to offer expert testimony.

APNs may also be qualified as expert witnesses regarding a physician's duty to supervise the APN. In *Harris v. Miller* (1994) CRNA William Hawkes administered anesthesia to Mrs. Harris while she was undergoing back surgery. Because the hospital did not employ any anesthesiologists, the anesthesia policy manual stated that the CRNAs functioned under the responsibility and supervision of the surgeons in the case.

The patient was obese and hypertensive, but CRNA Hawkes did not order an electrocardiogram. Additionally, he interpreted the patient's chest X-ray as normal, missing the patient's enlarged heart. He also failed to confirm correct placement of the endotracheal tube by checking for bilateral breath sounds, then attributed the patient's blood pressure drop during induction as a normal response to the nitrous oxide and Ethrane. The blood pressure continued to drop and the pulse rate increased, but CRNA Hawkes attributed these vital sign changes to pain, and administered high doses of Demerol and Innovar while continuing the Ethrane. The patient remained hypotensive and tachycardic throughout the procedure, but the CRNA did not advise the surgeon of these vital signs.

Although the average blood loss for the procedure was 100 cc's, Mrs. Harris lost approximately 400 cc's of blood. The surgeon, Dr. Miller, ordered the CRNA to transfuse the patient, but it was another 40 minutes before he did so. Although the patient continued to bleed, Dr. Miller never asked CRNA Hawkes about the patient's vital signs. The blood pressure continued to drop to a systolic of 70, but the CRNA still did not notify the surgeon of the hypotension. He also failed to reduce the anesthesia or increase the percentage of oxygen.

Despite the dangerously low blood pressure, CRNA Hawkes administered Demerol. When the systolic blood pressure was 40, he administered Neo-synephrine, but the vital signs continued to deteriorate. Only when there were no discernable pulse or blood pressure did the CRNA notify the surgeon of the problem. Mrs. Harris was resuscitated but had suffered neurological damage. Postoperative X-rays revealed that the endotracheal tube placement was such that only the right lung was being ventilated. Mrs. Harris and her husband brought a medical malpractice lawsuit against the hospital, Dr. Miller, and CRNA Hawkes.

At trial, the plaintiffs claimed Dr. Miller was negligent in supervising CRNA Hawkes. The Court excluded the expert testimony of CRNA

Sandra Privatte, who would have testified for the plaintiffs that: (a) Nurse Hawkes needed supervision in ascertaining that there was a medical crisis and in deciding what remedial measures should be taken, and (b) Dr. Miller had a duty to provide such supervision. The jury returned a verdict in Dr. Miller's favor and the plaintiffs appealed. The standard of care needed to be established by other practitioners in the particular field or by experts equally familiar and competent to testify to that limited field of practice. Stating that CRNA Privatte was not familiar with the standards of care for orthopedic surgeons and was, therefore, unqualified to testify as an expert witness, the Court of Appeals upheld the trial court.

The plaintiffs then appealed to the Supreme Court of North Carolina. Mr. Harris claimed that CRNA Privatte was fully qualified to testify and the exclusion of her testimony had prevented him from proving Dr. Miller's negligence. The claim against Dr. Miller was that he failed to adequately supervise CRNA Hawkes. CRNA Privatte testified that she was knowledgeable about what a CRNA can do without supervision. She was also knowledgeable about the manner in which surgeons supervise CRNAs.

The Supreme Court of North Carolina reasoned that the surgeon had agreed with the hospital to supervise the CRNAs assigned to his cases. CRNA Privatte was competent to testify regarding CRNA Hawkes' need for supervision in responding to a medical crisis. CRNA Privatte was also competent to testify as to Dr. Miller's duty to provide such supervision. In holding that she should have been permitted to do so, the Court reversed the verdict and remanded the case for a new trial.

When the subject matter falls distinctly within the realm of one profession, statutory mandates or the court may limit expert testimony to members of that profession. In *Sullivan v. Edward Hospital* (2004) plaintiffs offered the testimony of a physician as an expert regarding the standards of practice for nurses. The trial court ruled that the testimony was inadmissible, as the physician was not competent to testify regarding nursing standards of care. This decision was upheld on appeal, and the plaintiff continued the appeal to the Illinois Supreme Court. Arguments similar to those in *Baylor* were offered, that physicians, by virtue of their experience in working with nurses and observing their practice, are qualified to offer opinions regarding nursing standards. The argument was made that, "[T]here is nothing which a nurse can do which a doctor cannot do" (*Sullivan v. Edward Hospital*, p. 120).

The Illinois Supreme Court did not agree with this reasoning, agreeing instead with The American Association of Nurse Attorneys (TAANA):

A physician, who is not a nurse, is no more qualified to offer expert, opinion testimony as to the standard of care for nurses than a nurse would be to offer an opinion as to the physician standard of care ....Certainly, nurses are not permitted to offer expert testimony against a physician based on their observances of physicians or their familiarity with the procedures involved. An operating room nurse, who stands shoulder to shoulder with surgeons every day, would not be permitted to testify as to the standard of care of a surgeon. An endoscopy nurse would not be permitted to testify as to the standard of care of a gastroenterologist performing a colonoscopy. A labor and delivery nurse would not be permitted to offer expert opinion testimony as to the standard of care for an obstetrician or even a midwife. Nor would a nurse be permitted to testify that, in her experience, when she calls a physician, he/she usually...responds in a certain manner. Such testimony would be, essentially, expert testimony as to the standard of medical care. (*Sullivan v. Edward Hospital*, pp. 120–121)

The Court also quoted scholarly publications regarding the practice of physicians testifying as experts for nursing standards:

By enacting the Nursing and Advanced Practice Nursing Act...the legislature has set forth a unique licensing and regulatory scheme for the nursing profession. As TAANA observes, under the nursing act, a person with a medical degree, who is licensed to practice medicine, would not meet the qualification for licensure as a registered nurse, nor would that person be competent to sit for the nursing license examination, unless that person completed an accredited program in nursing. (*Sullivan v. Edward Hospital*, p. 122)

Physicians often have no first-hand knowledge of nursing practice except for observations made in patient care settings. The physician rarely, if ever, teaches in a nursing program, nor is a physician responsible for content in nursing texts. In many situations, a physician would not be familiar with the standard of care or with nursing policies and procedures which govern the standard of care. Therefore, a physician's opinions would not be admissible in jurisdictions which hold the expert must be familiar with the standard of care in order to testify as an expert. An example of a common situation which gives rise to allegations of nursing negligence occurs when a nurse fails to follow the institutional "chain of command" in reporting a patient condition to a physician who subsequently refuses to attend to the patient condition. It is unlikely that a physician would be familiar with the policy and procedure involved in handling such a situation. It is as illogical for physicians to testify on nursing standard of care as it would be for nurses to testify about medical malpractice. E.

Beyer & P. Popp, *Nursing standard of care in medical malpractice litigation: The role of the nurse expert witness,* 23 J. Health & Hosp. L. 363, 365 (1990). (*Sullivan v. Edward Hospital,* p. 121)

Although jurisdictions disagree on whether physicians may testify as experts regarding nursing standards of practice, the general consideration is whether or not the subject matter is sufficiently within the witnesses' training and knowledge to allow for a meaningful and reliable opinion. Absent statutory requirements, the admissibility of the testimony of a particular expert witness may depend less on whether or not he or she is a member of the same profession, and more on whether the allegations in the complaint involve issues within the expertise of the witness.

In *McElhaney v. Harper-Hutzel Hospital* (2006), a lawsuit claimed that the negligent actions of a nurse midwife caused an infant to suffer mental retardation and other impairments. The plaintiffs submitted affidavits of merit from obstetrician/gynecologists. (An affidavit or certificate of merit is a procedural requirement in many jurisdictions that requires the plaintiff, when filing a malpractice suit, to submit an affidavit from an expert licensed in the same profession as the defendant. The affidavit states that the affiant has been fully and fairly informed of the facts of the case and in the affiant's opinion, there is merit to the complaint. If the plaintiff does not meet all the procedural requirements for the affidavit or certificate of merit, the case may be dismissed.)

The hospital argued that the case should be dismissed because the physician affidavits of merit were defective. Regardless of whether the experts could establish that the injuries were caused by the midwife, they argued that they were not qualified to offer testimony regarding the standards of practice for nurse midwifery. Michigan law required an expert witness to devote a majority of his or her professional time to the active clinical practice *of the same health profession* as the defendant. The Michigan Court of Appeals agreed that to qualify to offer testimony regarding the appropriate standard of practice or care of the nurse midwife, plaintiff's experts must practice in "the same health profession" as the nurse midwife:

> Nurse midwives are licensed to practice under MCL 333.17211 certified under MCL 333.17210. Dr. Zack and Dr. Berke, however, are obstetricians/gynecologists who are physicians under the Public Health Code definition, MCL333.17001 (1)(c). These experts, therefore, do not qualify to testify regarding the standard of care applicable to defendant's nurse midwife. (*McElhaney v. Harper-Hutzel Hospital,* p. 496)

Although there is jurisdictional variation in expert witness requirements for nursing standards regarding duty and breach, there is little
debate that causation experts must be physicians. Whether or not the
negligence alleged caused the plaintiff's injury generally requires specialized knowledge and expertise beyond the scope of nursing, even at the
advanced practice level. In explaining to the jury how the departure
from standards caused the injury, the expert is offering diagnostic
impressions. Because the offer of expert testimony on causation is the
rendering of a medical diagnosis, it is considered to be within the
specialized knowledge of medicine.

In *Talmore v. Baptist Hospitals* (2006), the plaintiff offered the expert
report of an NP regarding a Stage II pressure ulcer. The report stated
the pressure ulcer developed as a result of the standard of care not
being followed. Texas statutes specified that only a physician could
testify as an expert witness on the causal element in a health care
liability claim. Accordingly, the Court stated, "Although qualified by
education, experience, or training, to express an opinion about the
nursing standard of care during Talmore's hospitalization at Baptist,
Nurse Practitioner Lindsay is disqualified by statute as an expert witness
on causation in this case."

Unlike the decision in *Talmore*, an exception may exist in some
jurisdictions for expert testimony regarding pressure ulcers. In *Gaines
v. Comanche County Medical Hospital* (2006), the patient brought a
malpractice action when he developed post-operative pressure sores on
his sacral area, feet, heels, and head. He offered an RN as his expert
witness. The defendants argued that the case should be dismissed because the plaintiff had not provided a physician to offer expert testimony.
The motion to dismiss was granted by the trial court, and the plaintiff
appealed. The Court of Civil Appeals recognized that the management
of pressure sores is a nursing responsibility and reversed the dismissal.
The defendants then appealed that reversal.

The Oklahoma Supreme Court agreed with the Court of Civil Appeals and remanded the case:

> The registered nurse's expertise makes her an appropriate professional to
> offer expert testimony concerning the practices of other nurses and the
> standard of care in the avoidance, treatment and cause of bed-
> sores....[W]ith the proper foundation, nurses should be qualified as ex-
> perts as to causation and as to treatment and cure of bedsores. In doing
> so, it recognized that such skin eruptions are "primarily a nursing prob-
> lem...nurses are experts." (*Talmore v. Baptist Hospitals*, fn 4)

Similarly, in *Freed v. Geisinger* (2009), an RN was used to testify as to the standard of care regarding the treatment and prevention of pressure wounds on an immobilized patient. She was not, however, allowed to testify that the departure from those standards resulted in the pressure sores. The trial court dismissed the suit, holding that because the RN was not a medical doctor, she was unqualified to offer testimony regarding causation. When the Superior Court reversed the trial court's dismissal of the case and remanded the case to trial, the defendants appealed to the Supreme Court of Pennsylvania.

The Supreme Court of Pennsylvania stated that state law permitted nurses to diagnose human responses to health problems, but prohibited nurses from providing medical diagnoses. That prohibition, however, did not necessarily mean nurses were prohibited from offering expert witness testimony, "[T]here is no language whatsoever in the statute to suggest that the principles governing the actual *practice* of nursing are applicable in the distinct *legal arena* of malpractice or negligence actions." The Court agreed that nurses may be qualified to offer expert testimony regarding the causation of pressure ulcers. In so reasoning, it affirmed the Superior Court's decision to send the case back to trial (*Freed v. Geisinger*, pp. 1202–1216).

Foreseeability

In addition to duty, breach, causation, and harm, the plaintiff may be required to demonstrate an element of foreseeability. The general principle of foreseeability is that a defendant will be held liable if his or her conduct is a substantial factor in bringing about harm to another. This is true even when the defendant did not foresee the extent of the harm or the manner in which it occurred (American Law Institute, 1980, § 435).[3] The court may determine that the defendant's actions are not the legal cause of the harm if it appears to the court that it would be highly extraordinary that the defendant's actions brought about the harm. The general standard is that a reasonable person of average intelligence would be able to anticipate the consequences of the defendant's actions.

In *Doege v. Sid Peterson Memorial Hospital* (2005), a patient filed suit after being sexually assaulted by a radiology technician during an ultrasound. The trial court dismissed the case against the hospital and the patient appealed. The hospital argued that the patient had not presented evidence that it could foresee the sexual assault. A nurse testified, however, that she had been previously sexually harassed by the radiology technician and had reported the incident prior to his assault of the patient. The supervisor had not reported the complaint, and the technician had not been counseled or disciplined. The Court of Appeals of Texas, Fourth District, San Antonio, reasoned that the hospital's failure to comply with its own harassment policies could be evidence that the hospital could have foreseen the sexual assault. Additionally, the hospital's actual knowledge of the technician's prior sexual misconduct raised the issue of foreseeability. The case was sent back to the trial court on that basis.

CAUSES OF ACTION

Claims against APNs are specialty-specific as found in Table 4.1. The most common allegations against all APNs, however, are complaints related to medication, treatment, and monitoring. Malpractice lawsuits frequently assert multiple claims. In addition to claims of medical negligence, plaintiffs may make several other allegations. Although not an exhaustive list, the most common causes of action include:

■ *Wrongful Death:* The estate of a deceased patient may bring suit, claiming the APN's departure from standards of practice caused the patient's death or caused injuries that subsequently lead to the patient's death. The statute of limitations for a wrongful death claim may be different than for medical malpractice.

■ *Lack of Informed Consent:* The patient claims to have suffered from a foreseeable complication of which he was not advised. Had he been so advised, he would not have consented to the treatment or procedure.

■ *Emotional Distress:* APNs can be accused of creating emotional distress intentionally or negligently. Claims of intentional infliction of emotional distress may fall under the state's intentional torts procedures and have a different statute of limitations than the associated malpractice claim. Claims of negligent infliction of emotional distress may fall under the state's negligence procedures.

■ *Loss of Consortium:* In addition to the loss of sexual relations, plaintiffs may also assert loss of companionship, loss of guidance and support, loss of society, or loss of other family benefits resulting from the malpractice. Some jurisdictions do not recognize these claims as a separate cause of action, but treat them as specific damages. The spouse of the injured party or other family member may assert these claims.

■ *Negligent Hiring/Negligent Supervision/Negligent Retention:* Employers have the responsibility to hire and supervise their employees.

NATIONAL PRACTITIONER DATA BANK 2006 ANNUAL REPORT

Table 4.1

Malpractice Reason	RN (Professional) Nurse*	Nurse Anesthetist	Nurse Midwife	Nurse Practitioner	Advanced Practice Nurse/Clinical Nurse Specialist*	Total
Anesthesia Related	137	973	1	10	1	1,122
Behavioral Health Related*	6	1	0	1	1	9
Diagnosis Related	253	17	43	267	2	582
Equipment or Product Related	60	6	0	6	0	72
IV or Blood Products Related	172	14	0	2	0	188
Medication Related	605	31	4	73	1	714
Monitoring Related	776	21	19	29	0	845
Obstetrics Related	428	7	483	32	1	951
Surgery Related	399	69	9	13	1	491
Treatment Related	761	36	36	148	6	987
Miscellaneous	227	6	1	13	0	247
All Reasons	3,824	1,181	596	594	13	6,208

* A professional nurse is an individual who has received approved nursing education and training who holds a BSN degree (or equivalent), an ADN degree (or equivalent), or a hospital program diploma, and who holds a state license as a registered nurse. This definition includes nurses who have advanced training as nurse midwives, nurse anesthetists, advanced practice nurses, etc.

Source: U.S. Department of Health and Human Services, Health Resources and Services Administration, Bureau of Health Professions, Division of Practitioner Data Bank. (2006). *National Practitioner Data Bank 2006 Annual Report* (p. 6). Retrieved April 30, 2010, from http://www.npdb-hipd.hrsa.gov/pubs/stats/2006_NPDB_Annual_Report.pdf

Health care institutions have a legal obligation to adequately screen potential new hires and monitor their performance. Failure to provide properly trained personnel may result in compensable patient harm.

■ *Falsified Records:* If the plaintiff believes the medical record has been altered, tampered with, or falsified, this may lead to an additional claim. Falsified business or medical records are extremely problematic, as they represent spoliation of evidence and undermine the credibility of the provider. All state boards identify falsification of medical records as professional misconduct, and such behavior also constitutes a federal crime.

THEORIES OF LIABILITY

Respondeat superior (Let the master answer)/Vicarious Liability): This is an agency theory holding that an employer is liable for the actions of its employees while acting within the course and scope of their employment. Because APNs are frequently employees, they act as agents of their employers and represent their interests. As such, the employers may be held responsible for their negligence. Because the employer is holding the APN out as a qualified professional, the employer has vicarious liability for the APN's actions.

Respondeat superior holds that the master is responsible for the actions of the servant. Hospitals, clinics, and school districts who hire APNs are clearly employers. For APNs working in collaborative practice structures with physicians, the employer–employee relationship may be less clear. APNs should seek legal guidance when entering into these contracts.

If the APN is acting outside of the organization's policies and procedures, or exceeding the allowed scope of practice within the institution, the employer may no longer be liable, as the APN is no longer acting in the interest of the employer, but is on what is called a *frolic and detour*. When the APN engages in activities that deviate from employer guidelines or regulations, he or she may bear the entire liability for those actions.

Ostensible Agency: Even when the APN has independent contractor status and is not an employee, the facility may be held responsible for the APN's negligence under a theory called ostensible agency (American Law Institute, 1980, § 429, p. 454).[4] The theory applies when the organization creates the appearance to the patient that it is supplying the provider. The patient's reasonable expectation is that the physician or APN is acting as an agent of the organization and functioning under its control. This patient belief supersedes whatever actual relationship exists between the organization and the provider. This is illustrated in a New York wrongful-death case, *Mduba v. Benedictine Hospital* (1976).

A hospital was sued after a patient died from motor-vehicle-accident injuries. The deceased's estate claimed the hospital was liable for the emergency department physician's failure to transfuse the patient in a timely fashion. The trial court dismissed the complaint, holding that the physician, Dr. Bitash, was an independent contractor. Because Dr. Bitash was not an employee of the hospital, the hospital could not be held liable for his actions. On appeal, the Third Department disagreed, finding that the emergency department physician was an employee.

Of greater importance, however, is the Court's reasoning that the employee–independent contractor distinction was irrelevant, because the hospital could be held responsible in either case:

> This is not a situation where the decedent engaged Dr. Bitash in defendant's hospital. The decedent entered the hospital for hospital treatment. The defendant hospital undertook to treat decedent for a charge and furnished the doctors and staff to render that treatment. Defendant having undertaken to treat decedent, which included both the necessary treatment and the furnishing of blood and other medicine needed in that treatment, was under a duty to do so effectively. Patients entering the hospital through the emergency room could properly assume that the treating doctors and staff of the hospital were acting on behalf of the hospital. Such patients are not bound by secret limitations as are contained in a private contract between the hospital and the doctor. Defendant held itself out to the public offering and rendering hospital services. (*Mduba v. Benedictine Hospital*, p. 453)

Corporate Liability: Health care organizations may have institutional liability for negligence. A 1965 Illinois case is generally credited for setting the precedent that a hospital may be held responsible for patient injuries. In *Darling v. Charleston Hospital* (1965), a college student was treated for a broken leg by the hospital's emergency room physician and nurses. When he ultimately underwent a below-the-knee amputation for gangrene, the father sued the hospital for failing to supervise its staff. The complaint alleged that the emergency room physician and the nursing staff failed to properly and timely assess the compromised circulation that ultimately led to the inability to save the leg. The claim against the hospital alleged inadequate supervision over its staff and physicians.

The Court was not persuaded by the hospital's defense argument that corporations do not practice medicine or nursing and therefore could not be held responsible: "[T]he Standards for Hospital Accreditation, the state licensing regulations and the defendant's bylaws demonstrate that the medical profession and other responsible authorities regard it as both desirable and feasible that a hospital assume certain responsibilities for the care of the patient" (*Darling v. Charleston Hospital*, p. 332).

Some jurisdictions adopt the thinking in *Darling* and allow negligence claims against health care organizations for improper credentialing, ineffective monitoring of physicians and employees, and inadequate staffing. Hospitals may be held accountable to injured patients for failures in administrative responsibilities. These jurisdictions recognize the changing nature of hospitals from mere buildings in which physicians work to sophisticated businesses and comprehensive health care centers. As such, they have the obligation to provide and monitor all aspects of health care.

Under a theory of corporate liability, the health care organization itself has a direct duty to the patient. The duty includes such things as providing proper equipment, premises safety, the promulgation and enforcement of policies and procedures, and the monitoring of physician and staff performance. Patients rely on the care they receive within a corporate structure. They believe the providers are working on behalf of the organization and come to the facilities thinking they will be cared for by the institution.

Other jurisdictions do not recognize such claims, holding that corporate obligations are determined by the legislature. In these jurisdictions, peer review regulations, accreditation standards, and specific statutory provisions dictate the organization's obligations, and the courts are reluctant to impose additional liability from civil suits. Although these jurisdictions may dismiss a claim under corporate liability theory for negligent credentialing or ineffective peer review procedures, they may still allow claims regarding general business practices. As such, health care organizations may still be liable for negligence in responsibility to the public for such things as wet floor signs, adequate lighting, elevator safety, or parking lot security.

Joint and Several Liability: Medical malpractice lawsuits frequently involve more than one individual defendant. Because a multitude of providers are involved in patient care, adverse outcomes may be attributed to the actions or inactions of many different parties. If the case goes to trial, the jury may return verdicts against some or all of the defendants. The theories of joint and several liabilities address the division of damage awards in cases with shared liability.

Joint Liability: In jurisdictions that use this system, each defendant is held individually responsible for the total amount of damages.

Several Liability: In jurisdictions that use this system, each defendant is responsible only for the portion of the total amount of damages that he or she created. In a hypothetical example, a nurse and a physician are both sued for a patient injury. If a jury determines that 60% of the cause of the injury was due to nursing negligence and 40% of the cause of the injury was due to medical negligence, the nurse will pay 60% of the award, and the physician the remaining 40%.

Joint and Several Liability: In this system, each defendant is responsible for the entire amount of the damages, regardless of the proportionate amount of liability for which he is responsible. In the example above, the nurse and the physician are each responsible for 100% of the award. If the nurse is unable to pay, the physician must pay the entire award. If the physician is unable to pay, the nurse must pay the entire amount. Whatever amount the one party cannot pay must be paid by the other party or parties. Jurisdictions that have adopted this system have done so to ensure that victims are fully compensated for their injuries. Jurisdictions that have not adopted joint and several liability systems, or who have limited, modified, or abandoned it, have done so in the interest of tort reform and out of concerns for unfairness.

The plaintiff can pursue the defendants individually or collectively, and may obtain separate judgments against them. If multiple defendants produce a single injury, they are all liable, however, the plaintiff may only receive compensation once.

In *Markley v. Oak Health Care Investors of Coldwater* (2003), a misdiagnosis in one facility led to a large-bowel resection and left-leg amputation. The patient was subsequently admitted to a nursing home. While in the nursing home, an NP increased the patient's intravenous rate, causing respiratory and cardiac arrest, from which the patient died. The family settled a wrongful death lawsuit against the first facility for $460,000. Of the $460,000, $220,000 was allocated for the wrongful death and $240,000 for conscious pain and suffering.

The family brought a separate suit against the nursing home and obtained a jury award of $300,000. The nursing home argued that it should only have to pay $80,000 of that award, because $220,000 of the $300,000 had already been paid by the first facility. (This is known as a "setoff" to ensure that a plaintiff only receives one recovery for his injury. The amount a plaintiff recovers from one defendant is "set off" against a subsequent verdict obtained against another defendant.)

The Court stated that the patient's death constituted a single, indivisible injury. Despite the fact that the family had brought distinct lawsuits, the hospital and the nursing home were jointly and severally liable for the wrongful death. The jury award of $300,000 against the nursing home had been partially paid by the hospital, and the nursing home needed to only pay the remaining $80,000.

PROFESSIONAL LIABILITY INSURANCE

Medical malpractice is an extremely complex, highly specialized, and enormously expensive area of negligence law. The APN who is sued requires the services of a skilled attorney to preserve rights and maximize the potential for a good outcome. Although the vast majority of malpractice suits are settled, dismissed, or result in defense verdicts, the emotional and financial costs of defending against the allegations can be considerable. In the event of a plaintiff's verdict, those losses may be catastrophic. "Going bare" or practicing without insurance coverage exposes the defendant in a lawsuit to personal expense and risk. Professional liability insurance can offset those expenses and provide protection for the provider faced with an expensive legal defense.

In the work environment, APNs can be held liable for their own practices, as well as for negligence in the monitoring and training of those under their supervision. APNs may also be included in claims against other providers with whom they practice, or in claims against the institutions in which they work. Outside of the work setting, APNs may be liable for negligence in offering advice or rendering emergency care. A personal professional liability insurance policy can provide legal representation when such suits occur. Additionally, a personal policy may provide licensure protection in the event that a complaint is made to the licensing board.

Because the insurance industry is regulated at the state level, premiums and coverage requirements differ by location. In most states, physicians must, by law, maintain malpractice insurance coverage. Some states also require APNs to be insured. APNs working within collaborative practice agreements with physicians should have their own coverage and not rely on the physician's policy as physician practice policies may not adequately cover the APN (*Elacqua v. Physicians' Reciprocal Insurers*, 2005). Privileges and credentials may be contingent upon having malpractice insurance, even when not required by statute.

Types of Policies

The two major types of insurance contracts are occurrence and claims made.

Occurrence policies are policies that cover claims arising from an event that occurred when the policy was in effect, regardless of when the claim is filed. Occurrence policies will cover claims that arise even after the policy has lapsed. They tend to be more expensive than claims-made policies. The amount the insured is covered for remains the same as when the policy was in effect.

Claims-made policies are policies that only cover claims involving events that occurred when the policy was in effect and that are reported during the terms of the policy. They tend to be less expensive, but "tail coverage" purchases may be necessary to cover claims that are reported after the policy term ends. The amount the insured is covered for is the amount the policy states at the time the claim is made.

Common Misconceptions

Some providers remain uninsured for reasons based upon misinformation or misconceptions about liability. The most commonly identified misperceptions are:

■ *Providers are more likely to be sued if they are insured than if they are uninsured.* Plaintiff's attorneys generally do not know the insurance status of the defendants at the time they are instituting suits on behalf of their clients. A decision to name someone in a suit is based upon the perception of that person's contribution to the patient's injury. Insurance information is exchanged as a part of the discovery process, and may influence the strategy to add or remove parties, but being uninsured will not prevent a provider from being sued.

If an injured patient believes he or she can prove that an APN departed from the standards of practice and that the departure caused compensable harm, it is unlikely that he will drop the suit against that APN simply because the APN is uninsured. A suit that goes forward against an uninsured APN creates expensive legal defense burdens and exposes the APN to the risk of a judgment for which he or she is personally responsible. Similarly, an injured patient will not name a person in a lawsuit simply on the basis of that person's insurance status. If the patient's attorney does not think a case can be made that a specific provider's departure caused an injury, he or she is unlikely to target that specific provider in the complaint. Contrary to the rhetoric about "frivolous" or "junk" lawsuits, plaintiff's attorneys bear the costs of litigation, and are only willing to do so when believing there is merit to the claim.

■ *Juries give higher awards to plaintiffs when the defendants are insured.* Juries do not have insurance information about any of the parties. The triers of fact are charged with determining whether the provider departed from standards and whether that departure caused harm. Insurance information is not probative of those inquiries, and is considered irrelevant and prejudicial.

■ *Providers with good practice skills do not get sued.* Human perfection is unattainable. Conscientious, highly skilled, and experienced professionals still make mistakes. Perpetual and flawless vigilance is not realistic, particularly when APNs work in dangerous systems. The majority of errors do not result in patient harm, but those errors that do create harm may be catastrophic. Good practice skills are not enough to keep patients safe. Moreover, even if the APN believes a complaint has no merit, the allegations must be defended against. Legal defenses are expensive, regardless of the ultimate outcome.

■ *Providers have immunity from lawsuits if they work in a governmental or charitable organization.* Many of the sovereign/governmental and charitable/religious immunities have been abolished or eroded. Those that do remain may be very narrowly construed. The immunity upon which the APN wishes to rely may only apply to discretionary duties (those involving judgment), and so, will not apply if the action for which the APN is being sued is considered to involve ministerial duties. Even if successful at establishing immunity, the APN litigating this argument will incur legal costs.

■ *There is no need to insure providers unless they have valuable assets to protect.* After a jury returns a plaintiff's verdict, the judge enters the jury's determinations as a court order. The defendant is then responsible for paying the award. If the defendant defaults on payment and the court judgment remains unsatisfied, the plaintiff may motion the court to enforce the judgment. Enforcement of the judgment may result in liens on property, seizure of assets and bank accounts, damage to credit, driver's license suspensions, wage garnishment, inheritance deductions, and additional legal expenses. More worrisome is the potential for an unsatisfied judgment to be considered professional misconduct by the licensing board.

■ *Employer policies ensure adequate protection.* Employer malpractice polices are written to protect the employer, not the employee. Employers may have vicarious liability for the actions of their employees while acting within the scope of their employment. They have insurance for that reason, not as an employee benefit. Lawyers representing the employers in a malpractice suit must do what is in the best interests of their clients, the employers. Acting in the best interest of the employer may result in actions that are adverse to the employee. Unless the interests of the employer and the APN are clearly harmonious, it may not be in the APN's best interests to be represented by counsel acting for the benefit of that employer.

When the employer and the APN are each named as codefendants, they may have divergent or competing interests regarding claims coverage, defense strategies, jury selection, or settlement of the case. Because an attorney cannot represent clients with conflicting interests, the APN needs separate representation and the undivided loyalty of his or her own counsel (Hytko, 2009). Additionally, employers may have the right to seek indemnification from their employees. (An indemnification suit is one in which a party who has suffered losses requests that another party assume the financial responsibility for that loss.) APNs must have their own liability coverage against these claims.

Employer policies only cover the employees while acting within the scope of their employment. The employer's insurance carrier may elect to not represent the APN who is accused of violating institutional policies and procedures or acting outside the scope of the employer's job description. Any suits that arise from actions not related to the work place will also not be covered by the employer's policy. Employer policies only cover malpractice. The APN who is reported to the board of nursing also needs legal representation. This gap in employer coverage leaves the APN without coverage in licensure defense actions.

Finally, many employers are self-insured and/or have shifted from occurrence to claims-made policies. Upon separating from the employer with a claims-made policy, the APN becomes uninsured. Liability protection ends when terminating employment. This creates a coverage lapse until the APN is re-employed or has a personal policy. For these and all the above-explained reasons, APNs are strongly advised to obtain and maintain individual professional liability insurance policies.

COLLATERAL IMPACT

APNs involved in lawsuits in which a settlement is reached, or a plaintiff's verdict is obtained, may be reported to data banks (U.S. Department of Health and Human Services, 2006). The Office of the Inspector General (OIG) may place the APN on an exclusion list, prohibiting the APN from directly receiving or being employed by a recipient of Medicaid and Medicare funding. Nursing boards may consider such lawsuits as evidence of unsafe practice and/or professional misconduct. For a discussion of data banks, nursing board actions, and OIG exclusion lists, refer to chapter 6 on licensure and regulation. A recent discipline forum in Texas revealed a foreseeable consequence of malpractice reform efforts. Texas passed caps on punitive damages in 2003. Since the caps went into effect, patients have sought redress by increasing their complaints to licensing boards.

REDUCING EXPOSURE

Interpersonal Skills

The APN who is perceived as competent, trustworthy, empathetic, and professional is significantly less likely to be sued than the APN who is perceived as impersonal, unapologetic, or less than forthcoming with information. Many patients will decide not to sue when presented with open disclosure of errors and/or a simple apology (Leape, 2005). APNs who are sued are in a better position to defend themselves if there is clear documentation of timely and honest discussions regarding errors. The traditional objection to apologizing to patients has been the concern that such apologies will be construed in court as admissions of liability (Wei, 2007). For this reason, some states have enacted apology laws that provide immunity for such discussions. Although further research is needed to determine whether such laws improve provider–patient relationships and deter lawsuits, APNs are certainly more sympathetic defendants when juries think they have apologized and accepted responsibility. Compassion, kindness, and respect are as essential as clinical competence in reducing liability.

Documentation

Lessons learned from the cases in this chapter suggest that APNs must carefully document all conversations with patients regarding consent, instructions, side effects of medications, the need for follow up, and pending diagnostics. Medical records should indicate all communication between providers and capture witnesses to any essential conversations. Charting should be consistent with institutional policies and procedures and indicate evidence-based practice. Discharge notes must include an assessment of the patient's condition and consistency with the APN/physician collaborative practice agreement.

Insurance

For all the reasons discussed above, APNs are strongly advised to carry their own professional liability insurance, independent of their employer's policy. APNs in collaborative practice agreements with physicians should be familiar with the partnership or practice's insurance policy to know whether they are listed insureds, and whether there are indemnity clauses. Personal malpractice policies may also provide representation for APNs who have not been named in lawsuits, but have been subpoenaed to testify as witnesses. Even when merely providing witness testimony, APNs should be represented by counsel to avoid inadvertently making statements against their own interest.

SUMMARY

A widely cited Institute of Medicine report, *To Err Is Human: Building a Safer Health System* (Institute of Medicine, 1999), centered attention on the issue of patient safety. The report estimated that medical errors cause 44,000–98,000 hospital deaths per year. These statistics are considered to be an underrepresentation of the problem (Center for Justice and Democracy, n.d.) Health care institutions and providers can only respond to these findings effectively by addressing the root causes of medical error. The traditional health care culture does not lend itself to the nonpunitive error reporting or analysis that is necessary for quality improvement. Its hierarchical structure and expectations of perfection in clinical practice do not allow providers to readily admit their mistakes. Guilt and shame further deter patient safety efforts and contribute to a culture of blame.

Misconceptions concerning malpractice liability divert attention and undermine efforts to improve delivery systems and practice patterns. If providers are focused on "tort reform" rather than true patient safety initiatives, medical error will remain unaddressed, as will the underlying reasons patients decide to sue them. "Reform" efforts must be directed toward encouraging disclosure and the reduction of medial error. Fears of liability constrain such efforts.

Despite pervasive rhetoric about litigious patients, the vast majority of APNs will never be involved in lawsuits. The professional and ethical responsibility to advocate for patients must take the form of timely disclosure, honest dialogue, and root cause analysis for system improvement. APNs cannot allow error reporting and analysis to be compromised by misguided fears of litigation. Ultimately, it is simply not possible to advocate for patients while simultaneously viewing them as potential adversaries.

KEY POINTS

1. Although it is possible to understand general concepts of malpractice and negligence, malpractice lawsuits are primarily litigated in state courts with considerable variation in statutes of limitation, procedures, statutory constructions, bodies of case law, and jurisdictional requirements.
2. The perception of liability risk far exceeds the reality, and that perception undermines patient safety as it erodes the provider–patient relationship and deters error reporting and analysis.
3. APNs can reduce their liability exposure by fostering trustworthy relationships with patients, practicing within institutional policies and collaborative practice agreements, using best practices in documentation, and embracing transparency.
4. Individual professional liability insurance policies can provide a measure of security for APNs that employer policies do not, including licensure representation and suits arising from outside of the workplace.
5. APNs have an ethical responsibility to challenge those deeply ingrained traditions in health care that demand perfection in practice and encourage silence for human error.

NOTES

1. Tex. Civ. Prac. and Rem. Code Ann. § 74.351(a)—any person who has brought a suit asserting a health care liability claim must, within 120 days of filing the claim, provide an expert report for each physician or health care provider against whom the claim is asserted. If the claimant does not provide an expert report as required, the trial court must, upon motion by the defendant, dismiss the claim with prejudice.
2. Restatement of the Law (2d) of Torts, § 328D. *Res Ipsa Loquitur:* It may be inferred that harm suffered by the plaintiff is caused by negligence of the defendant when:
   - the event is of a kind that ordinarily does not occur in the absence of negligence
   - other responsible causes, including the conduct of the plaintiff and third persons, are sufficiently eliminated by the evidence

■ the indicated negligence is within the scope of the defendant's duty to the plaintiff.

It is the function of the court to determine whether the inference may reasonably be drawn by the jury, or whether it must necessarily be drawn. It is the function of the jury to determine whether the inference is to be drawn in any case in which different conclusions may reasonably be reached.

"[U]nder the doctrine of *res ipsa loquitur*, negligence may be inferred where [1] the injuring instrumentality is shown to be under the management or exclusive control of the defendant or his servants and [2] the accident is such as in the ordinary course of things does not happen if those who have management of the injuring instrumentality use proper care" (Restatement of the Law of Torts, § 328D).

3. Restatement of the Law (2d) of Torts, § 435. Foreseeability of Harm or Manner of Its Occurrence: (a) If the actor's conduct is a substantial factor in bringing about harm to another, the fact that the actor neither foresaw nor should have foreseen the extent of the harm or the manner in which it occurred does not prevent him from being liable, and (b) the actor's conduct may be held not to be a legal cause of harm to another where after the event and looking back from the harm to the actor's negligent conduct, it appears to the court highly extraordinary that it should have brought about the harm.

4. Restatement of the Law (2d) of Torts, § 429, page 454: "One who employs an independent contractor to perform services for another which are accepted in the reasonable belief that the services are being rendered by the employer or by his servants, is subject to liability for physical harm caused by the negligence of the contractor in supplying such services, to the same extent as though the employer were supplying them himself or by his servants."

REFERENCES

American Law Institute. (1980). *Restatement of the law (2d) of torts*. St. Paul, MN: West Publishing.

Baker, T. (2007). *The medical malpractice myth*. Chicago: University of Chicago Press.

Boothman, R., Blacknull, A., Campbell, D., Commiskey, E., & Anserson, S. (2009, January). A better approach to medical malpractice claims? The University of Michigan experience. *Journal of Health & Life Sciences Law, 2*(2). Retrieved August 14, 2009, from http://www.med.umich.edu/news/newsroom/Boothman%20et%20al.pdf

Center for Justice and Democracy. (n.d.). *The degree and cost of medical malpractice—Key findings of the National Academy of Sciences Institute of Medicine*. Retrieved August 16, 2009, from http://www.centerjd.org/archives/issues-facts/MB_IOM.pdf

General Accounting Office. (2003, June). *Report to congressional requesters, medical malpractice insurance multiple factors have contributed to increased premium rates, at 28.* Retrieved August 14, 2009, from http://www.gao.gov/new.items/d03702.pdf

Hunter, R. (2007, December 17). *Report of J. Robert Hunter, Director of Insurance, Consumer Federation of America to Joanne Doroshow, Executive Director, Center for Justice and Democracy on the current New York State medical malpractice situation.* Retrieved August 14, 2009, from http://www.centerjd.org/archives/states/newyork/CJDHunterAnalysis pdf.pdf

Hunter, R., Cassell-Stiga, G., & Doroshow, J. (2009, July 22). *True risk: Medical liability, malpractice insurance and health care.* Retrieved April 11, 2010, from http://www.centerjd.org/air/TrueRiskF.pdf

Institute of Medicine. (1999). *To err is human: Building a safer health system.* Washington, DC: National Academies Press.

Keeton, W., Dobbs, D., Keeton, R., & Owen, D. (1984). *Prosser and Keeton on the law of torts* (5th ed.). St. Paul, MN: West Publishing.

Leape, L. (2005). Understanding the power of apology: How saying "I'm sorry" helps heal patients and caregivers. *National Patient Safety Foundation Newsletter, 8,* 3.

Mello, M. (2006a, January). *Understanding medical malpractice insurance—A primer.* Harvard School of Public Health, research synthesis report no. 8. Retrieved August 16, 2009, from http://www.rwjf.org/pr/synthesis/reports_and_briefs/pdf/no10_primer.pdf

Mello, M. (2006b, May). *Medical malpractice: Impact of the crisis and effect of state tort reforms.* Harvard School of Public Health, research synthesis report no. 10. Retrieved August 14, 2009, from http://www.rwjf.org/pr/synthesis/reports_and_briefs/pdf/no10_rese archreport.pdf

National Association of Insurance Commissioners. (2009). *Countrywide summary of medical malpractice insurance, 1991–2004.* Retrieved April 11, 2010, from http://www.naic.org/documents/topics_Med_Mal_premiums_loss.pdf.

North Carolina Advocates for Justice. (2009, May 5). *Medical malpractice lawsuits in North Carolina, 1998–2008.* Retrieved August 14, 2009, from http://www.mountainverdict.com/mountain-verdict-blog-lawyer-attorney/209-surprising-medical-malpractice-statistics.html

Schauffler, R., LaFantain, R., Strickland, S., & Rafferty, W. (2006). *Examining the work of state courts, 2005: A national perspective from the court statistics project.* Retrieved August 14, 2009, from http://207.242.75.69/cgi-bin/showfile.exe?CISOROOT=/ctad min&CISOP TR=412

Schmitt, C. (2008, June 20). *U.S. News and World Report.*

Smarr, L. (2005, April 7). *Physician Insurers Association of America, testimony before the House Judiciary.* Retrieved August 18, 2009, from http://www.ihatoday.org/issues/liability/talk/smarrtest.pdf

Studdart, D., Mello, M., Gawande, A., Gandi, T., Kachalia, A., Yoon, C., et al. (2006, May 11). Claims, errors, and compensation payments in medical malpractice litigation. *New England Journal of Medicine, 354*(19), 2024–2033. Retrieved August 14, 2009, from http://www.hsph.harvard.edu/faculty/michelle-mello/files/litigati on.pdf

United States Department of Health and Human Services. (2006) *National Practitioner Data Bank 2006 annual report.* Retrieved August 14, 2009, from http://www.npdb-hipdb.hrsa.gov/pubs/stats/2006_NPDB_Annual_Report.pdf

Wei, M. (2007, Winter). Doctors, apologies, and the law: An analysis and critique of apology laws. *Journal of Health Law, 9*(4), 300–304.

TABLE OF CASES

5

Labor and Employment Issues

EDITH ANN BROUS

It is apparent much of the ANA Code...is focused on care. This focus on care has led some nurses to be less prepared to understand issues (e.g., finances and policy) and processes like conflict resolution. When we lack understanding of these fundamental issues, it is almost unavoidable to lapse into a vision of oneself and one's colleagues as powerless victims in a senseless system.

—*Kathleen O. Williams*

INTRODUCTION

Advanced-practice nurses (APNs) may be employees, independent contractors, business partners, or solo practitioners. The statutes and regulations, employer and business responsibilities, tax obligations, benefit eligibility, and worker rights that impact APN practice, therefore, depend on the practice setting and the nature of the APN's association with it. In the United States, worker classifications are defined by the Internal Revenue Service (IRS). Courts base their interpretations of these classifications on the relationship between the worker and the business.

Graduate curricula that focus solely on the clinical aspects of nursing practice fail to prepare APNs with the business and financial education that are essential to successful practice in those advanced roles. To compete in the health care marketplace, APNs must understand the economic, political, ethical, and legal environment in which they practice. Although such a discussion is beyond the scope of this book, this chapter will discuss employment and labor laws in general, as well as particular APN workplace issues.

EMPLOYMENT RELATIONSHIPS

Employees

APNs who work in hospitals, clinics, schools, or other businesses may be employees. The IRS considers an APN an employee if the facility in which the APN works maintains behavioral and financial control over the APN. Behavioral control is the right to direct or control how the work is performed. Considerations include how, when, and where the work is performed, what equipment is used, what assistants are hired to help the APN, and where supplies and services are purchased (Internal Revenue Service, 2008). A critical consideration is the level of instruction or training provided to the APN. Financial control is the extent to which the business directs or controls the financial and business elements of the APN's practice. Considerations include the APN's investment in the practice setting, reimbursement for expenses, the method of payment to the APN, and the APN's market opportunity to provide services and incur profit or loss.

In addition to behavioral and financial control, courts analyze the type of relationship between the APN and the organization. Facts suggesting that the APN is an employee include the payment of benefits (insurance, pension, paid leave, vacation time) and payroll deductions for income tax, Medicare and unemployment insurance taxes, and Social Security. Courts will also consider the intention of the parties to continue working together, the nature of the work performed, and the existence of a written agreement or employment contract. APNs will be considered employees if the organizations in which they work have the right to control what the APN does, where the APN works, and how the APN works.

Employers may have vicarious liability for the negligence of their employees. This liability is premised on the employer's control over the practice and performance of its workers. Employers must make tax and Social Security payments on behalf of their employees. Employees are covered under the labor and antidiscrimination laws, as discussed in the following text.

Employment-at-Will

APNs working within traditional employer–employee structures are parties to what is termed the employment-at-will doctrine. In the absence of contractual language to the contrary, the APN–employer relationship continues indefinitely at the will of both parties. Either party may end the relationship at any time. A notable exception to the employer's ability to lawfully terminate an APN is when the termination violates antidiscrimination laws. An employer also may not terminate an APN for refusing to violate the law or public policy. In some states, employers who terminate APNs to avoid paying accrued benefits may be subject to liability for breach of what is called a *covenant of good faith and fair dealing*. A notable exception to the APN's right to leave employment at any time is when to do so would endanger the public or constitute patient abandonment.

Contractual Employment

APNs may have individual employment contracts with the organizations in which they work. Such contracts are not open-ended as in the employment-at-will structure, but contain specific dates for starting and ending employment. The employer and the APN are bound by the terms of the agreement, and either party may be liable to the other for breaching those terms. APNs may also be represented by unions, in which case APNs are parties to collective bargaining agreements.

Independent Contractors

APNs working in collaborative practice partnerships, assigned to facilities through employment agencies, or in private practice may be considered independent contractors. APNs who function as independent contractors are responsible for meeting their own tax obligations (income tax and self-employment tax). To be considered an independent contractor, the facility in which the APN works must only have the right to control the result of the APN's work, but not the means and methods of accomplishing that work. Independent contractors are not entitled to employee benefits. As such, vacation, pension, health benefits, sick time, and malpractice insurance are generally not provided. APNs working as independent contractors are not included in the organization's workers compensation insurance.

Because organizations do not have control over the means by which independent contractors practice, they may not have liability for the negligence of APNs functioning as independent contractors. Employers may classify workers as independent contractors, rather than employees, to obtain tax and negligence liability advantages. Labor law requirements such as minimum wage and overtime pay do not apply to independent contractors. The IRS analyzes 20 different factors to determine whether an APN is an employee or an independent contractor, as summarized in Table 5.1 (Internal Revenue Service, 2009).

Determination of Worker Classification

Correct worker classification is essential to the organization for tax purposes, and to the APN for benefit purposes. The landmark case establishing this importance is *Vizcaino v. US District Court for W.D. of Wa* (1999). The Microsoft Corporation supplemented its regular employee workforce with freelancers and temporary agency workers. The IRS conducted an audit and determined that Microsoft had misclassified 483,000 freelancers as independent contractors when, in fact, they were employees. Microsoft then offered some of these workers positions as employees. Most of the freelancers, however, were told to convert to temporary agency worker status or leave Microsoft. Although the agency "payrolled" the converted workers, all other aspects of the worker/Microsoft relationship remained unchanged.

The freelancers brought a class action suit against Microsoft, alleging that they had met the definition of "employee" but had been denied benefits, because Microsoft had classified them either as independent contractors or as employees of their agencies (referred to as "temps"). Specifically, they had been denied the opportunity to participate in Microsoft's Savings Plus Plan (SPP) and employee stock purchase plan (ESPP). Microsoft argued that, although the workers met the legal definition of employees, they had signed independent contractor agreements expressly providing that they were responsible for their own benefits. The Court found that they were entitled to ESPP participation during the time they had worked as temps. Whether or not the workers were employees of Microsoft or of the agencies was deemed irrelevant. The Court found that Microsoft, not the agencies, had maintained control over recruitment, training, duration of employment, and work assignments.

Vizcaino held that Microsoft exercised or retained the right to exercise direction over the services provided by the temp workers and it was that control, not who payrolled the workers, that determined the status of those workers as Microsoft employees. As such, they were

Table 5.1

DISTINCTIONS BETWEEN EMPLOYEES AND INDEPENDENT CONTRACTORS

EMPLOYEE	INDEPENDENT CONTRACTOR
1. **Instructions/training:** Organization has the authority to require APN's compliance with instructions about when, where, and how to work	APN determines when, where, and how to work
2. **Instructions/training:** Facility controls the manner in which the APN works, provides training regarding facility policies and procedures	APN practices independently
3. **Integration:** APN's services essential to the business of the facility	APN's services not necessary to the business of the facility
4. **Services rendered personally:** APN personally performs the work	APN may assign the work to others
5. **Hiring, supervising, and paying assistants:** APN may hire, supervise, or pay other workers subject to the employer's terms	APN may hire, supervise, or pay other workers pursuant to contractual terms
6. **Continuing relationship:** APN may work for the same facility for many years	APN is hired for a particular job with no expectation of a continuous relationship
7. **Set hours of work:** Facility schedules the APN	APN controls the work schedule
8. **Full-time status:** APN works full time for the organization	APN works when and for whom he or she wants
9. **Work done on premises:** APN works in employer's facility	APN may work off-site
10. **Order or sequence set:** APN does things in the order prescribed by the organization	APN performs the work in whatever order or sequence he or she chooses
11. **Reports:** APN must submit periodic oral or written reports	APN not required to submit reports
12. **Payment:** APN paid in regular intervals/pay periods	APN paid by assignment
13. **Payment of expenses:** APN's business expenses paid by employer	APN responsible for own business expenses
14. **Furnishing of tools and materials:** Facility provides materials, tools, equipment	APN may provide all necessary supplies

(continued)

Table 5.1 *(continued)*

EMPLOYEE	INDEPENDENT CONTRACTOR
15. **Significant investment:** APN does not have significant investment in the facility	APN may have significant investment in the facility
16. **Profit or loss:** APN's performance and decisions do not affect profit/loss potential	APN's performance and decisions may affect profit/loss potential
17. **Working for more than one organization at a time:** APN generally works only for one organization	APN may work for many different organizations
18. **Making services available to the general public:** APN's services are provided to the organization's patients	APN may own his or her own businesses and make services available to the general public
19. **Right to discharge:** APN can be terminated at any time	APN can only be terminated pursuant to contractual terms
20. **Right to resign:** APN can resign at any time	APN may be contractually bound to complete a specific term of employment

entitled to participate in the ESPP program. Microsoft was fined ($751 million) and a settlement was reached, in which Microsoft agreed to deposit $96,885,000 into a fund to be distributed to the class action members. Additionally, Microsoft changed its staffing and worker-classification practices, hiring more than 3,000 of the class members as W-2 employees who were eligible to participate in employee benefits (*Vizcaino v. Microsoft Corp.*, 2002, p. 1046). The case clarified the law regarding temporary worker classification. Workers who would previously have been misclassified as contingent workers, and therefore ineligible for benefits, now may receive the benefits associated with full-time employment (*Vizcaino v. Microsoft Corp.*, 2002, p. 1040).

Similar decisions were made against FedEx for $26.8 million (*Pittsburgh Business Times*, 2008), The *Orange County Register* for $22 million (Gittleson, 2009), American Airlines for $325,000 (*DiFiore v. American Airlines, Inc.*, 2009), and Time Warner for $5.5 million (Time Warner, 2000). The variety and complexity of APN–employer relationships make it difficult to generalize or predict court decisions, but there is a general presumption that the worker in an employee versus independent contractor dispute is an employee. It is the employer's burden to demonstrate independent contractor status.

Vizcaino is relevant to APNs working through staffing agencies. In the traditional employer–employee relationship, the APN works as an agent (the servant) of one organization (the master). *Vizcaino* held that a person may be the servant of two masters. Although staffed and payrolled through an agency, the APN may be considered an employee of the recipient of his or her services. The APN's service to the one does not necessarily involve abandonment of service to the other. The APN may still be legally defined as an employee of the organization even though a "triangular relationship" exists between the APN, the agency, and the organization. In a negligence lawsuit, the APN may be considered the servant of the organization, of the agency, or of both. The determining factor is the level of control the organization has over the APN's practice.

APNs' RIGHTS AS EMPLOYEES

Workplace rights are established by federal, state, and local laws. When there is conflict between state and federal law, the federal law generally prevails. An exception exists when the state laws are more stringent or protective than the federal laws. The individual states and territories may enact their own laws, but they must be consistent with the minimum requirements of the federal laws. State-specific regulations are promulgated and enforced by various agencies and interpreted by the courts.

Department of Labor

Fair Labor Standards Act of 1938

The Fair Labor Standards Act (FLSA, 1938) was enacted in 1938. It governs wages, hours, overtime, recordkeeping, and child-labor standards, as well as setting the minimum wage. FLSA specifically provides protections for triangulated relationships, referred to as coemployment or joint employment relationships. In situations in which employers share the APN's services, in which one employer acts in the interest of another employer in relation to the APN, or in which employers share control of the APN, both employers may be responsible for compliance with FLSA's requirements. APNs assigned to facilities through staffing agencies may be considered joint employees of both the facility and the agency.

Employers are required to pay workers at least the minimum wage for all hours worked. Additionally, workers must be paid at least 1½ times their regular pay rates for all hours worked in excess of 40 hours per week. Records must be kept for each worker, including the employee's full name, Social Security number, address, birth date (if younger than 19), sex, occupation, workweek and workday hours, wage basis, hourly pay rate, total straight time and overtime earnings, wage additions and deductions, total wages per pay period, and dates of payments and pay periods (FLSA, 1938). The FLSA's requirements only apply to "nonexempt" employees. "Exempt" employees are those who meet three tests related to how much the employee is paid (at least $23,000 annually), how the employee is paid (salaried basis), and what kind of work the employee performs (such as executive, administrative, or professional duties) (FLSA, 1938, 29 C.F.R. 541). APNs may be classified under the FLSA as nonexempt employees and thus be entitled to overtime pay, as illustrated in *Belt v. EmCare, Inc.* (2005).

EmCare employed physician assistants (PAs) and nurse practitioners (NPs) to provide emergency room care in 20 states. The PAs and NPs were paid straight time on an hourly basis (not salaried) for all hours worked, including those over 40 hours per week. The PAs and NPs performed the same job duties: obtaining histories, performing physical examinations, ordering diagnostics, making preliminary diagnoses, and providing treatment in collaboration with physicians. Fifty-nine PAs and 20 NPs brought a suit for back wages and liquidated damages, claiming EmCare had violated the FLSA in not paying them at the overtime rate after 40 hours a week. EmCare argued that the PAs and NPs were exempt as "learned professionals," notwithstanding the fact that they were paid on an hourly basis and not salaried (FLSA, 1938, 29 C.F.R. 541.314).

Under the regulations, employees may be exempt from the FLSA's requirements if they meet the definition of "learned professionals:"

> To qualify for the learned professional exemption, an employee's primary duty must be the performance of work requiring advanced knowledge in a field of science or learning customarily acquired by a prolonged course of specialized intellectual instruction.

This primary duty test includes three elements:

1. The employee must perform work requiring advanced knowledge
2. The advanced knowledge must be in a field of science or learning
3. The advanced knowledge must be customarily acquired by a prolonged course of a specialized intellectual instruction [FLSA, 1938, 29 C.F.R. 541.314(a)].

The court held that PAs and NPs must be paid on a salaried basis to be exempt as learned professionals. Because EmCare paid them on an hourly basis, they were not exempt. On appeal, EmCare argued that PAs and NPs fell under an exception to the salary basis rule. They argued that because NPs and PAs exercise a great degree of independent discretion and have a large amount of advanced training, they were exempt as bona fide "white collar" professionals. The exception applies to "an employee who is the holder of a valid license or certificate permitting the practice of law or medicine or any of their branches and who is actually engaged in the practice thereof," and is referred to as the "Exception for physicians, lawyers, and teachers" (FLSA, 1938, 29 CFR 541.314). EmCare interpreted this exception to include PAs and NPs.

The regulations expressly excluded registered nurses (RNs) from the salary basis rule, but did not address NPs or PAs. The Fifth Circuit, therefore, needed to determine whether PAs and NPs were practicing medicine or "related professions which merely service the [medical] profession" (*Belt v. EmCare, Inc.*, 2006, p. 413). The Court held that the Department of Labor (DOL) was the agency entrusted by Congress to define who was eligible for professional exemption to the salary requirement. Despite "higher barriers to entry and the increasing sophistication of their practice," the DOL had not included PAs and NPs along with physicians, attorneys, and teachers. As such, PAs and NPs were "nascent" professions in need of the FLSA's protection. As nonexempt employees, the PAs and NPs were protected "against the threat of the evil of overwork as well as underpay" (*Belt v. EmCare, Inc.*, 2006, p. 417).

Family and Medical Leave Act of 1993

The Family and Medical Leave Act of 1993 (FMLA, 1993) applies to businesses with 50 or more employees [FMLA, 1993, § 2611 (2)(B)(ii)], and also considers coemployment situations and temporary workers. The agency may be designated as the primary employer and the facility as the secondary employer. As primary employers, agencies provide leave to eligible APNs. As secondary employers, the facilities continue to use the APN's services upon return from leave. Secondary employers cannot interfere with the APN's rights under the FMLA, and may be held liable for violations of the Act when doing so (FMLA, 1993, § 2617).

The Act requires employers to provide an eligible employee up to 12 weeks of unpaid leave from the job for a "serious health condition" that renders the employee unable to perform the essential functions of the position. Eligible employees are those who have worked for the employer for 12 months, and who have worked a minimum of 1,250 hours in the 52 weeks prior to starting the FMLA leave [FMLA, 1993, § 2601(b)(1)-(2)]. Eligible employees may elect, or an employer may require, that vacation time, sick time, or personal time be substituted for part of the 12-week period.

Upon return from FMLA leave, the employer must return the employee to the previous position or an equivalent position—one that is identical in pay, benefits, working conditions, privileges, status, duties, and responsibilities, and one that requires the same skill, responsibility, and authority [FMLA, 1993, § 2614(a)(1)(B)]. The APN returning from FMLA leave does not have more reinstatement rights than if such leave were not taken. The employer may demonstrate that the APN would not have been kept in a particular position even if he or she had been continuously employed, because the position was eliminated or the APN would have been terminated for non-FMLA reasons.

APNs who bring suit against their employers for FMLA violations must show that they are eligible employees under the Act, that the facilities in which they work are covered employers under the Act, that they were entitled to leave under the FMLA, that they provided the employer with adequate notice of the intent to take leave, and that they were denied benefits to which they were entitled, were treated less favorably than employees who had not requested FMLA leave, or that an adverse decision was made because the APN sought protection under the FMLA.

In *Staples v. Parkview Hospital, Inc.* (2009), a nurse was terminated after 15 years in her position at the hospital. The reason given for her termination was that she violated the hospital's strict antiharassment policy by asking sexual questions of a coworker. The nurse brought suit, claiming that the real reason she was fired was because she was about to take time off pursuant to the FMLA. She claimed that other nurses had made similar sexual comments, and that she was terminated because she had identified that she was going to undergo carpal tunnel and bariatric surgery. She also claimed the termination was retaliation for exercising her FMLA rights.

The hospital sought to have the case dismissed, arguing that she had not been entitled to leave and that she had failed to provide adequate notice of her intent to take FMLA leave. The Court believed there was a question as to whether or not the nurse had given her supervisors enough information to trigger the hospital's obligation to investigate whether she was entitled to FMLA leave. Once an employee establishes a prima facie case, the burden shifts to the employer to produce a nondiscriminatory reason for its actions. (A plaintiff establishes a prima facie case when producing sufficient evidence to raise a presumption of fact or to establish the fact in question unless rebutted.) The hospital argued that the decision to terminate the nurse was completely unrelated to her intent to take FMLA leave. It maintained that she was terminated for creating a sexually hostile work environment.

Once an employer offers a nondiscriminatory reason for its actions, the burden shifts back to the plaintiff to show that the reason offered by the employer is merely a pretext. The employee can refute the employer's reason by establishing that it is baseless, that the reason was not the true reason for the action, or that the reason would have been insufficient to motivate the employer to take that action. In this case, the nurse was able to provide enough evidence to question whether her coworkers were offended by her comments to create the hostile work environment claimed by the hospital. She was also able to offer sufficient evidence that she may have been treated differently than other employees who did not ask for FMLA. The Court held that she had provided sufficient evidence to question whether the nondiscriminatory reason given by the hospital was valid or pretextual. The Court was presented with two different interpretations of what led to her termination. What really happened, then, was a question of fact. Because the facts are determined by juries, not judges, the Court denied the hospital's motion to dismiss and sent the case back to the trial court.

When APNs take leave under FMLA, they have the right to return to their positions or a position of equivalent benefits, pay, and terms as the position they left. In *Vlahos v. Schroeffel* (2006), Theresa Vlahos was a senior NP in a Complimentary and Alternative Medicine Unit (CAM) when she took medical leave in April of 2001. Human Resources (HR) responded to her request for an extension of the leave by informing her that she had to exhaust her sick accruals, which were sufficient to cover absences through September of 2001.

Upon her return to work in October of 2001, Vlahos signed a form requesting FMLA leave for a chronic condition and requested clarification of her sick accruals. HR informed her that she had used her sick accruals and was not eligible for FMLA. HR argued that because she had not been working between April and October of 2001, she had not worked a minimum of 1,250 hours during the 52 consecutive weeks prior to when her FMLA leave would begin. The Court found that the employer could not evade responsibility for compliance to the FMLA if Vlahos was qualified for FMLA leave from April to October of 2001, but was using sick time during that period. The hospital was not permitted to use its sick time policy to render Vlahos ineligible for FMLA benefits.

When Vlahos returned to work, she was assigned to work in Pre-Admission Testing (PAT), as the CAM unit had been eliminated. Vlahos filed suit, claiming that the hospital violated the FMLA by not restoring her to the same or equivalent position. She contended that the PAT position was significantly different from her position in the CAM unit. Additionally, Vlahos claimed the hospital had been under an obligation to determine whether she was eligible for FMLA leave beginning in April of 2001.

The Court also determined that a reasonable jury could find that the CAM and PAT positions were not equivalent, as the role of an NP in CAM was different from the role of the NP in PAT. Vlahos no longer had the ability to see patients in follow-up visits or maintain ongoing relationships with patients, as she had in the CAM. In the PAT, Vlahos was only able to see patients once for a history and physical prior to surgery. Because the PAT was not service-based, as was the CAM, she could not see patients post-operatively, nor could she write prescriptions or treat the patients. Because there was a question as to whether the positions were equivalent, the Court denied the hospital's motion to dismiss the case.

National Labor Relations Act of 1935

In 1935, Congress enacted the National Labor Relations Act (NLRA, 1935), also referred to as the Wagner Act, to protect the rights of both employees and employers. The intent of the Act was to encourage collective bargaining (NLRA, 1935, § 157) and make certain management and labor practices [NLRA, 1935, § 158(a)(b)] unlawful. Such practices were thought to compromise the national economy through their damaging impact on interstate commerce (NLRA, 1935, § 1.151). The Act guaranteed employees the right to conduct secret ballot elections for organizing, and provided employees with the right to bargain collectively. Employees could choose representatives to represent them in negotiations over wages and working conditions.

The National Labor Relations Board (NLRB) was created to administer the Act [NLRA, 1935, § 3.153(a)] and, along with the courts, enforces its provisions. The NLRA gave workers the right to join labor unions, bargain collectively, and strike. It prohibited employers from refusing to bargain in good faith with the unions, or from discouraging union membership. Specific provisions apply to the health care industry [NLRA, 1935, § 213(a)]. The definition of employer included private, nonprofit hospitals. The NLRA has been amended several times as the political climate toward labor has changed.

Labor Management Relations Act/ Taft-Hartley Act of 1947

The Labor Management Relations Act (LMRA), more commonly known as the Taft-Hartley Act, was enacted in 1947 as an amendment to the NLRA. It was a response to Congressional concerns about corruption within the unions, and provided for DOL oversight of union finances and election activity. The Taft-Hartley Act also reflects Congressional Cold War concerns about the political power of unions, in that it prohibited the union from making campaign contributions to federal politicians. Additionally, the Act prohibited Communist party membership, actually requiring union leaders to sign non-Communist affidavits.

The LMRA was also a response to concerns that union strikes were hampering the economy. As such, it defined and prohibited unfair labor practices by labor unions, such as jurisdictional, wildcat, and sympathy strikes, secondary boycotts, and closed shops. For a definition of these and other terms, refer to Exhibit 5.1. Nonprofit hospitals were excluded under the Act, removing NLRA protection for nurses in such institutions. The Taft-Hartley Act also added "supervisor" to those excluded by the NLRA. Labor organizations have viewed the Taft-Hartley Act as antilabor, and have campaigned for its repeal.

Labor Management Reporting and Disclosure Act/Landrum-Griffin Act of 1959

A Congressional perception that unions were under the influence of organized crime resulted in the Labor Management Reporting and Disclosure Act/Landrum-Griffin Act of 1959 (LMRDA). The Act further regulated union financial activities in response to concerns about collusion, corruption, violence, and the diversion of funds, and it outlined fiduciary obligations (LMRDA/Landrum-Griffin Act, 1959, 29 U.S.C. § 501) and requirements for public reporting (LMRDA/Landrum-Griffin Act, 1959, 29 U.S.C. § 435). A 3–13-year waiting period was imposed on former convicts between the date of prison release to holding union office (LMRDA/Landrum-Griffin Act, 1959, 29 U.S.C. § 504). A bill of rights guaranteed union members the ability to conduct secret elections,

Exhibit 5.1

Common Terminology in Labor and Employment Law

Closed shops: Collective bargaining agreements only permitting employers to hire members of a particular labor organization.

Professional employee: (a) Any employee engaged in work (i) predominantly intellectual and varied in character as opposed to routine mental, manual, mechanical, or physical work; (ii) involving the consistent exercise of discretion and judgment in its performance; (iii) of such a character that the output produced or the result accomplished cannot be standardized in relation to a given period of time; (iv) requiring knowledge of an advanced type in a field of science or learning customarily acquired by a prolonged course of specialized intellectual instruction and study in an institution of higher learning or a hospital, as distinguished from a general academic education or from an apprenticeship or from training in the performance of routine mental, manual, or physical processes; or (b) any employee, who (i) has completed the courses of specialized intellectual instruction and study described in clause (iv) of paragraph (a), and (ii) is performing related work under the supervision of a professional person to qualify himself to become a professional employee as defined in paragraph (a). (29 U.S.C., Title 29, Chapter 7, Subchapter II).

Secondary boycott: Worker/labor pressure or coercion on a third party to stop doing business with a company that is the subject of a labor action.

Strikes: Concerted mass refusals to work or work stoppages.

Jurisdictional strike: A union's refusal to work in protest of the employer's assignments to nonunion members or members of a different union.

Sympathy strike: Workers striking in support of other strikers.

Wildcat strike: Workers unofficially striking without the labor organization's authorization or sanction.

Supervisor: Any individual having authority, in the interest of the employer, to hire, transfer, suspend, lay off, recall, promote, discharge, assign, reward, or discipline other employees, or responsibly to direct them, or to adjust their grievances, or effectively to recommend such action, if in connection with the foregoing the exercise of such authority is not of a merely routine or clerical nature, but requires the use of independent judgment. (29 U.S.C., Title 29, Chapter 7, Subchapter II).

Unfair labor practice: Interfering with, restraining, or coercing employees in the exercise of their rights under the NLRA.

Employer unfair labor practice examples: Discrimination in hiring or retaining employees or in terms and conditions of employment to impact labor organization membership, refusal to bargain collectively with employee representatives.

Union unfair labor practice examples: Discrimination against an employee for reasons other than failure to pay dues, refusal to bargain collectively with the employer, encouraging, inducing or engaging in unlawful picketing or strikes, forcing the employer to recognize or bargain with a labor organization that has not been certified as the representative of the employees.

Union shops: Organizations that require newly hired employees to join a union as part of the collective bargaining agreement.

speak freely, hold meetings, and be disciplined in accordance with due process requirements (LMRDA/Landrum-Griffin Act, 1959, 29 U.S.C. § 411). The Act strengthened parts of the Taft-Hartley Act, further restricting union activities related to secondary boycotts. Reflecting continuing Cold War concerns, the Act prohibited former Communist party members from holding union office for a 3–13-year period after resigning from the Communist party (LMRDA/Landrum-Griffin Act, 1959, 29 U.S.C. § 504). Union leaders were limited to 3–5-year terms (LMRDA/Landrum-Griffin Act, 1959, 29 U.S.C. § 481). Labor unions have regarded the Landrum-Griffin Act as further governmental encroachment into labor union authority.

Health Care Amendments of 1974

Nonprofit hospital exceptions were repealed, again allowing nurses employed in these institutions to be covered under the NLRA [Health Care Amendments, 1974, 29 U.S.C. § 2(14)]. Specific provisions were written to protect patients and prevent care disruption. Although nurses now had the right to strike, unions representing nurses were required to give employers 10 days notice prior to the scheduled strike date [Health Care Amendments, 1974, 29 U.S.C. § 213(a)]. Mediation was to be used, and cooling-off periods of 60 days could be ordered by mediators if patient safety was considered an issue (Health Care Amendments, 1974, 29 U.S.C. § 202–203).

Congress was concerned that multiple bargaining units would increase costs and create potential disruptions in patient services. In enacting the 1974 Amendments, therefore, it included an admonition to the NLRB: "[D]ue consideration should be given by the Board to preventing proliferation of bargaining units in the health care industry" (S. Rep. No. 766, p. 5, United States Code Cong. & Ad. News at 3950; H. Rep. No. 1051, 93d Cong., 2d Sess. 6, 1974). The NLRB responded to this directive by analyzing bargaining unit disputes on a case-by-case approach, which resulted in considerable litigation. In 1989, the NLRB adopted a rule limiting bargaining units within acute care hospitals to eight categories (NLRB, 1989, CFR § 103). Psychiatric hospitals and nonacute health care facilities continued to be litigated on a case-by-case basis.

To request an election for a bargaining unit to represent nurses or APNs, the union must file a petition and demonstrate that at least 30% of the workers are interested in being so represented. The NLRB determines whether the bargaining unit is appropriate. A "community of interests" standard was traditionally used, in which the NLRB evaluated employee qualifications, wages, training, work hours, supervision, working conditions, areas of practice, interaction with other employees, and other factors.

An example of the "community of interest" analysis is presented in *McLean Hospital Corporation and Massachusetts Nurses Association* (1993). The Massachusetts Nurses Association (MNA) petitioned to represent all RNs within this psychiatric facility. The hospital argued that separate bargaining units for nurses would compromise the therapeutic milieu and patient care, strain employee relationships, and create logistical problems in scheduling treatment team meetings. McLean wanted the smallest bargaining unit to be an all-professional unit, representing all licensed professionals. MNA argued that the RNs constituted a discrete group with distinct interests requiring separate representation. Because psychiatric hospitals were not included in the eight bargaining unit limit rule, the NLRB analyzed the dispute within a community-of-interests framework. It considered the team approach, as well as the substantial interaction and contact between the RNs and other professionals in mental health care settings.

The NLRB was not persuaded by the hospital's argument that an all-RN unit would compromise the team approach to patient care. The NLRB reasoned that RNs were the only professionals required to work 24 hours a day and 7 days a week. Additionally, RNs were the only professionals regularly required to work overtime. RNs were administratively segregated and managed by other nurses. RNs constituted a distinct labor market that was not interchangeable with other workers. "Although all professional employees have certain working conditions, personnel policies, and benefits in common, the RNs share other unique working conditions, interests, and benefits which distinguish them sufficiently from the remaining professionals to warrant separate collective bargaining" (*McLean Hospital Corporation and Massachusetts Nurses Association*, p. 1112).

The "community of interests" test was replaced with a "disparity of interests" test in *NLRB v. St. Francis Hospital of Lynwood* (1979). In this case, the union filed an election petition for a bargaining unit of all RNs. The hospital argued that the bargaining unit should represent all professionals, not just RNs. The hearing officer ruled that RNs comprised an appropriate unit and ordered an election, which the union won. The union brought an unfair labor charge when the hospital then refused to bargain with the union. The NLRB ruled against the hospital, ordered it to bargain with the union, and sought court-ordered enforcement of its order.

The Court analyzed the NLRB's "community of interests" factors for RNs, such as 24-hour duties, administrative segregation, and licensing requirements, and disagreed with the NLRB. The "community of interests" analysis had created an NLRB per se policy that RN units were appropriate. This was thought to be inconsistent with the legislative history of the NLRA. A policy broadening, rather than narrowing, bargaining units failed to give due consideration to the congressional directive to avoid proliferation:

> [W]e have a problem in fully appreciating the Board's...rationale...that because registered nurses have a "community of interests" they are entitled to a separate unit. While the community of interest standard may be decisive in other industries, it is not entirely controlling for the health care industry in the present context...Congress has made it clear that the Board must view evidence of traditional factors in the context of the stated Congressional policy of preventing proliferation of bargaining units in the health care field. (*NLRB v. St. Francis Hospital of Lynwood*, 1979, p. 418)

The Court stated that the NLRB should consider not the similarities among employees in the same job classification, but the "disparity of interests" among employee classifications. "[B]y including nonprofit hospitals within the Act, Congress sought to extend to hospital employees effective labor rights. By focusing on the disparity of interests between employee groups which would prohibit or inhibit fair representation of employee interests, a balance can be made between the congressional directive and the employees' right to representation" (*NLRB v. St. Francis Hospital of Lynwood*, 1979, p. 419). A separate bargaining unit for RNs could only be justified if "sharper than usual" differences existed regarding wages, hours, and working conditions. Separation would be justified if dissimilarity of interests among other providers precluded combination in the same bargaining unit.

The NLRB attempted to reduce the amount of litigation regarding the issue of appropriate bargaining units by exercising its rulemaking authority. In 1989, final rules and regulations were adopted, establishing eight distinct bargaining units within acute care hospitals (NLRB, 1989, § 103.30). The NLRB rule stated that, in the absence of extraordinary circumstances, the only appropriate bargaining units were RNs, physicians, professionals other than nurses and physicians, technical employees, skilled maintenance employees, business office clerical employees, guards, and nonprofessional employees other than technical employees, skilled maintenance employees, business office clerical employees, and guards. The rule was challenged, but upheld by the United States Supreme Court (USSC) (*American Hospital Assn. v. NLRB*, 1991).

As the role of the APN has evolved since the 1989 NLRB rule, some certified registered nurse anesthetists (CRNAs) have petitioned for distinct bargaining units. *Fair Oaks Anesthesia Associates v. NLRB* (1992) is an example. Despite NLRB certification of the Fair Oaks CRNA Association as the exclusive representative of the CRNAs, Fair Oaks Anesthesia Associates (the employer) refused to bargain with the association. The NLRB ruled that refusal to bargain was an unfair labor practice and ordered the employer to bargain. The employer stated that the Fair Oaks CRNA Association was an inappropriate bargaining unit, as the bargaining unit should be composed of both the CRNAs and the physician anesthesiologists.

Fair Oaks Anesthesia Associates argued that a "disparity of interests" test would find insufficient differences between the CRNAs and the physician anesthesiologists to warrant separate bargaining units. The employer further argued that allowing the CRNAs to have their own bargaining unit would create the fragmentation and proliferation of bargaining units that the NLRB's rule sought to avoid. The union argued that the "community of interests" test should be used because there were only two job classifications to be considered. The Fourth Circuit found that the CRNAs were a distinct classification, sharing a strong community of interests among themselves. The Court also found material and significant differences in the terms and conditions of employment applicable to the CRNAs and the physicians. "Sharper than usual interests" existed in wages, benefits, scheduling supervision, qualifications, and expectations of partnership to justify the separate bargaining unit. The separate CRNA bargaining unit was, therefore, appropriate.

The NLRA applies to employees, but not to independent contractors. The NLRB has traditionally held that temporary workers supplied by agencies are jointly employed by the agencies and the facilities to which they are assigned. Those contingent workers have traditionally been included in the same bargaining unit as the facility's regular workers for community of interest reasons. In 2004, however, the NLRB held that inclusion of both temporary and permanent workers in the same bargaining unit (referred to as multiemployer units) was only permissible with the consent of both employers.

In *Oakwood Care Center* (2004), employees of Oakwood, a long-term residential care facility, along with employees supplied to Oakwood by a staffing agency, petitioned for a bargaining unit. The NLRB determined that "[S]olely employed employees and jointly employed employees are employees of different employers and...their inclusion in the same bargaining unit creates a multiemployer unit" (*Oakwood Care*

Center, 2004, p. 662). The NLRB held that such combined units of solely employed and jointly employed employees were permissible only with the parties' consent. The petition was denied because neither Oakwood nor the staffing agency had consented to bargaining with each other in a multiemployer unit.

The *Oakwood* decision has been criticized as compromising contingent workers. In modern health care settings, many employers use temporary workers for economic reasons. The agencies furnishing these workers may not truly be employers in the traditional sense. Because *Oakwood* disregards this joint employment dynamic, employees in such triangulated relationships are less able to improve working conditions and fully exercise their rights. Labor proponents (Schiffer, 2005), and the dissenting opinion in the case (*Oakwood Care Center*, 2004, pp. 663–670), determined the decision failed to recognize the rights of employees who are employed by one entity but controlled by another. It effectively gives employers veto power over union representation, which frustrates union organizing. CRNAs are particularly likely to be in employment situations affected by the decision in this case.

There are circumstances in which APNs may belong to the same bargaining unit as RNs, even when employed by different entities. This is illustrated in *The NewYork Presbyterian Hospital and New York State Nurses Association* (2009). NPs were represented at NewYork-Presbyterian Hospital (NYPH) by the New York State Nurses Association (NYSNA). The collective bargaining agreement (CBA) had a standard provision that, "[E]xcept for certification, training or experimentation and emergencies, registered nurses who are outside of the bargaining unit will not routinely or consistently perform those clinical duties normally performed by members of this bargaining unit" (*The NewYork Presbyterian Hospital and New York State Nurses Association*, 2009, p. 3).

In 2004, a group of NPs on the payroll of the Columbia University School of Medicine were observed providing services to NYPH patients. NYSNA filed a grievance, claiming that NYPH had hired NPs in a nonunion capacity to do bargaining unit work. The remedy sought was to make the NPs union positions. NYPH denied the grievance, advising NYSNA that the NPs were Columbia University (CU) employees and not under the hospital's control or governed by the hospital's policies and procedures. The union then filed charges with the NLRB against the hospital and the university. NYSNA argued that the hospital and the trustees of the university were a single employer that had hired NPs under different terms and conditions of employment than those in the CBA.

The regional director of the NLRB referred the dispute to arbitration. CU advised NYPH and NYSNA that as a nonsignatory to the CBA, it would not participate as a party in the arbitration, nor would it be bound by any arbitration decisions. NYSNA issued a subpoena to the hospital seeking documents between NYPH and CU related to the NPs, such as names, titles, assignments, dates of hire and termination, job descriptions, salary, shifts, wages, and benefits. The documents were not produced and the university did not appear in the arbitration. The hospital claimed it did not have the information NYSNA requested, and the arbitrator did not issue a ruling on the subpoena. The union requested an adjournment and went to the NLRB to obtain the information.

NYSNA filed a complaint alleging that NYPH refused to provide information identifying the university NPs. The NLRB was not persuaded that NYPH did not have the information, reasoning that the NPs would have submitted the information for privileging purposes, whether employed by the hospital or the university. The NLRB was also not persuaded by NYPH's argument that it was not required to furnish information about non-bargaining unit employees. Although the union sought information about non-union employees, it did so for the purpose of processing a grievance in administering the CBA:

> The Union's grievance in this case related to the alleged performance of bargaining unit work by certain individuals whom [NYPH] asserts are not really its own employees. Nevertheless, the Union had obtained reliable information that these individuals (who happen to be on the payroll of Columbia University) performed work as nurse practitioners (a bargaining unit position) with the hospital for patients who are being treated in the hospital. From any objective point of view, these people are doing the same type of functions, in the same place for the same people, under the same supervision, under the same State laws and pursuant to the same type of privileges as the nurse practitioners who are directly employed by the [hospital]. (*The NewYork Presbyterian Hospital and New York State Nurses Association*, 2009, p. 7)

The NLRB ruled that refusing to furnish the information to NYSNA was an unfair labor practice in violation of NLRA, and ordered NYPH to provide the requested information.

APNs as "Supervisors"

The NLRA definition of employee explicitly excludes "any individual employed as a supervisor" [NLRA, 1935, § 2(3)], which is, in turn, defined as "any individual having authority, in the interest of the employer, to hire, transfer, suspend, lay off, recall, promote, discharge, assign, reward, or discipline other employees, or responsibly to direct them, or to adjust their grievances, or effectively to recommend such action, if in connection with the foregoing the exercise of such authority is not of a merely routine or clerical nature, but requires the use of independent judgment" [NLRA, 1935, § 2(11)]. Because they are not covered by the Act, supervisors can be excluded from the bargaining units, do not have the right to form, join, or assist unions, nor can they vote in NLRB elections or circulate petitions.

Although the statutory definition of supervisor includes the use of "independent judgment," it does not prescribe the degree of discretion required to be considered "independent judgment." The NLRB interpretation of "independent judgment" has led it to conclude that in some cases, the nurses are supervisors, although in others, they are not.

Professionals, however, are expressly included as employees entitled to the protections of the Act. An ambiguity exists when nurses, particularly APNs, may be defined as both supervisors and as professionals. In *NLRB v. Health Care and Retirement Corp.* (1994), the NLRB held that four licensed practical nurses (LPNs) were not supervisors, as claimed by the employer. The NLRB applied three tests to determine whether employees were supervisors:

1. Does the employee have the authority to engage in one of the 12 listed activities (hire, transfer, suspend, lay off, recall, promote, discharge, assign, reward, or discipline other employees, or responsibly to direct them, or to adjust their grievances, or effectively to recommend such action)?
2. Does the exercise of that authority require the use of "independent judgment"?
3. Does the employee hold the authority "in the interest of the employer"?

In this case, the NLRB reasoned that the LPNs' direction of aides was not authority exercised "in the interest of the employer," but was the exercise of professional judgment incidental to the treatment of patients. The Sixth Circuit agreed with the employer that the LPN direction of aides was in the interest of the employer and reversed the NLRB, holding that the LPNs were supervisors. The Court stated that Congress needed to carve out an exception for nurses if it did not want them to be considered supervisors.

A divided (five of the nine justices) United States Supreme Court (USSC) agreed that the LPNs were supervisors and affirmed the Sixth Circuit, reasoning that the NLRB had created a false dichotomy between patient care and acts taken in the interest of the employer:

> Patient care is the business of a nursing home, and it follows that attending to the needs of the nursing home patients, who are the employer's customers, is in the interest of the employer. (*NLRB v. Health Care & Retirement Corp.*, 1994, p. 577)

> The welfare of the patient, after all, is no less the object and concern of the employer than it is of the nurses. (*NLRB v. Health Care & Retirement Corp.*, 1994, p. 580)

It is important to note that four of the nine justices dissented, arguing that the term "supervisor" was being construed too broadly, such that most professionals would be excluded from the protections of the NLRA: "[T]he Court's opinion has implications far beyond the nurses involved in this case. If any person who may use independent judgment to assign tasks to others or direct their work is a supervisor, then few professionals employed by organizations subject to the Act will receive its protections" (*NLRB v. Health Care & Retirement Corp.*, 1994, p. 598).

NLRB v. Health Care and Retirement Corp. was followed by another important case in 2001. In *NLRB v. Kentucky River Community Care* (2001), the labor union petitioned the NLRB to represent a group of employees at a residential care facility. The facility objected to the inclusion of RNs, claiming that, as supervisors, they were excluded from the Act. The NLRB rejected the facility's designation of RNs as supervisors, reasoning that the nurses did not use "independent judgment" when directing other workers. It found nursing direction of less-skilled employees to reflect "ordinary professional or technical judgment" in accordance with the employer's standards, and ordered the facility to bargain with the union.

The Sixth Circuit refused to enforce the NLRB's order, rejecting its interpretation of "independent judgment." A divided USSC again affirmed the Sixth Circuit's holding that the nurses were supervisors. The Court disagreed with the NLRB's distinguishing two different kinds of judgment ("independent" and "ordinary professional or technical"), finding that it introduced a categorical exclusion not found in the text of the Act. As in *NLRB v. Health Care and Retirement Corp.*, the dissent argued that the interpretation of "supervisor" was too broad. The dissenting justices argued that "supervisor" should be restricted to those personnel with genuine management prerogatives, and not applied to minor supervisory employees, such as the nurses in this case (*NLRB v. Kentucky River Community Care*, 2001, pp. 723–724).

Since *Kentucky River*, labor organizations have expressed concern that expansion of the term "supervisor" will result in the exclusion from unionization of professional workers. The Courts and the NLRB itself have been divided enough to suggest that the issue is not resolved. Unless there is legislative intervention, the matter will continue to be litigated in the Courts.

In *Hospital General Menonita v. NLRB* (2004), the union filed a petition with the NLRB seeking to represent the hospital's RNs. The hospital opposed, arguing that the RNs were supervisors, therefore excluded from the NLRA. The NLRB decided that the RNs were not supervisors and ordered an election, which the union won. The NLRB certified the union as the exclusive bargaining agent of the RNs. The union filed an unfair labor practice complaint when the hospital refused to enter into contract negotiations with the union. The NLRB found that the hospital had committed an unfair labor practice by refusing to bargain and ordered it to do so.

The First Circuit stated that RNs could not be considered supervisors unless they met all three of the *Kentucky River* tests discussed previously. The mere fact that employees periodically instruct other employees does not make them supervisors. The Court held that the discretion of the RNs in this case was constrained by physicians' orders and institutional protocols, negating their supervisory discretion. Detailed orders and regulations could serve to reduce employee discretion below what would be necessary to deem them supervisors. As such, the Court ordered that the NLRB's order to the hospital to enter into negotiations with the union be enforced.

APNs may theoretically have more difficulty being included in the NLRA's protections under this *Hospital General Menonita* theory. Although institutional protocols may still be viewed as reducing the APN's supervisory discretion, the "constraints" of physicians' orders are less likely to apply to practitioners who themselves write orders, prescribe, and order diagnostic tests. The Courts and the NLRB will continue to approach the issue within the context of case-by-case analysis. As the political climate changes, the composition of those bodies changes as well, rendering uncertainty and inconsistency in the APN's right to engage in collective bargaining.

In 2007, House Resolution (HR) 1644 (2007–2008) was introduced into the 110th Congress, but it was never voted on to become law. The

"Re-Empowerment of Skilled and Professional Employees and Construction Tradesworkers" (RESPECT) Act would have reversed the decisions expanding the definition of "supervisor" by eliminating the terms "assign" and "responsibly direct" from the NLRA's definition of supervisor. RESPECT would also have required that workers spend the majority of their workday in a supervisory role to be deemed a supervisor. Nursing organizations and organized labor supported the bill. Hospital and management industries opposed it, arguing that it would constrain their ability to manage their staff.

EQUAL EMPLOYMENT OPPORTUNITY COMMISSION

Agency or temporary workers may bring discrimination claims. An APN, whether a full-time employee or a contingent worker, has the right to be hired, assigned, and treated in a nondiscriminatory manner. As with the DOL, coemployment liability may exist for employers under the Equal Employment Opportunity Commission (EEOC).

Title VII of the Civil Rights Act of 1964

Title VII is a federal law that makes it unlawful for the employer to discriminate against a person on the basis of race, color, religion, sex, or national origin. The employer who refuses to hire, discharges, or otherwise discriminates against a person on this basis is in violation of the Act. Employment practices that are considered unlawful under the Act are those that limit, segregate, or classify employees or applicants in a manner that deprives them of opportunities, or adversely affects their status as employees on the basis of those protected classifications [Civil Rights Act of 1964 [CRA, 1964], § 703(a)-(b)]. State and local antidiscrimination laws may be more inclusive or more stringent than the federal law, but analysis of complaints is generally within a Title VII framework. This is illustrated in *Hammond v. Cty. of Los Angeles* (2008).

Yvonne Hammond was a 62-year-old nursing instructor for the Medical Staff Development (MSD) unit of the Los Angeles County Sheriff's Department. She taught 7–10 classes per month, totaling 25–30 hours per week. Shortly after Betty Brennan was assigned as the MSD supervisor, she asked Hammond to accept a position as a staff nurse with a lower salary, telling her she was too old to stay in the classroom. Brennan then hired younger staff nurses to teach. In response to a new nursing director's instructions, Brennan scheduled Hammond to teach 12–20 hours a week. Hammond was the only African American among the four instructors. Brennan selectively monitored Hammond's classroom performance, but not that of the other three Philippine instructors. Brennan made derogatory remarks about African Americans and stated that she didn't understand Hammond because she was probably speaking "Ebonics."

When Hammond complained to Brennan's supervisor, Brennan became agitated and threatening. Hammond complained to another supervisor, and an investigation revealed that her complaints were founded. Hammond then filed a complaint under the state's antidiscrimination law, alleging race discrimination, age discrimination, and retaliation.

The trial court granted the County's motion to dismiss the complaint and Hammond appealed. The Court of Appeals for the Second Circuit noted discrimination claims must be proved circumstantially by means of the *McDonnell Douglas* test. The test comes from a 1973 civil rights case, *McDonnell Douglas Corp. v. Green*, in which the USSC noted that direct evidence of intentional discrimination is rare, and explained the means by which circumstantial proof may be offered (*McDonnell Douglas Corp. v. Green*, 1973). To prevail, Hammond needed to demonstrate that: (a) she was a member of a protected class, (b) she was qualified for the position she sought or was performing competently in the position she held, (c) she suffered an adverse employment action, and (d) some other circumstance suggested a discriminatory motive.

The Court concluded that Hammond had provided sufficient evidence to suggest that the adverse employment action may have been based on racial animus. As in FMLA cases, if the plaintiff establishes a prima facie case, the burden then shifts to the defendant to demonstrate that the adverse action was taken for a nondiscriminatory motive. Whether Brennan's actions constituted racial harassment and/or were motivated by age discrimination were issues of fact for a jury. The Court reversed the dismissal and reinstated the case. At trial, the employer would need to offer race-and age-neutral reasons for Brennan's actions. Hammond would then need to prove that the reason offered was pretextual.

Americans With Disabilities Act of 1990

The American With Disabilities Act (ADA) was enacted to prohibit discrimination against disabled or handicapped individuals in the workplace. The Act "prohibits private employers, state and local governments, employment agencies and labor unions from discriminating against qualified individuals with disabilities in job application procedures, hiring, firing, advancement, compensation, job training, and other terms, conditions, and privileges of employment" and applies to employers with 15 or more employees, employment agencies and labor organizations. (United States Equal Employment Opportunity Commission, 2009). In response to concerns that courts were defining the Act's terms too narrowly, the Act was amended in 2008 to make it easier for individuals seeking protection under the Act to establish that they had disabilities (ADA Amendments, 2008).

Employers may not discriminate against employees or applicants on the basis of disability or handicap, nor may they retaliate against employees who have filed discrimination claims. APNs who think they have been discriminated against may file a complaint with the EEOC. To claim disability discrimination, the APN must show that he or she has a qualifying disability or is disabled within the meaning of the ADA, that he or she is a qualified individual and able to perform the essential functions of the job, and that the adverse action was due, at least in part, to the disability.

Disabilities are physical or mental impairments that substantially limit one or more life activities. Considerations include the nature and severity of the impairment, the duration or expected duration of the impairment, and the real or expected permanent or long-term impact of the impairment. Employers are required to make reasonable accommodations to employees or applicants with disabilities, unless doing so would impose "undue hardship" in the operation of the employer's business.

As with all discrimination cases, the *McDonnell Douglas* test is used. The APN must establish a prima facie case of disability discrimination. The burden then shifts to the employer to set forth a legitimate and nondiscriminatory reason for the adverse action. The APN then must refute the proffered reason as pretextual. The EEOC recognizes that certain impairments present different challenges for health care settings. Additionally, health care providers are at risk of particular workplace hazards, such as needle sticks, latex allergies, musculoskeletal injuries, and shift-related injuries (United States Equal Employment Opportunity Commission, 2007).

Rehabilitation Act of 1973

Like the ADA, the Rehabilitation Act of 1973 prohibits discrimination on the basis of disability. The Act specifically addresses such discrimination against employees working in the federal government, and applies to employers receiving federal funds or contracting with the federal government. As with ADA complaints, an APN alleging discrimination under the Act must demonstrate that he or she has a qualifying disability or is disabled within the meaning of the ADA, that he or she is a qualified individual and able to perform the essential functions of the job, and that the adverse action was due, at least in part, to the disability.

Age Discrimination in Employment Act of 1967

Congress enacted the Age Discrimination in Employment Act (ADEA) to address disadvantages found by older persons in retaining employment. Arbitrary age limits imposed by employers excluded able candidates and created hardship among older workers. The Act makes it unlawful for employers to refuse to hire, discharge, or otherwise discriminate against anyone on the basis of age. Prohibitions against age discrimination apply to labor organizations, as well. The Act makes it unlawful to exclude or expel any members on the basis of age. Neither the employer nor the labor organization may limit, segregate, or classify employees in any manner that adversely affects compensation, terms, conditions, or privileges of employment or opportunities. As the nursing workforce ages, age discrimination cases are likely to become more prominent. The employer must be capable of articulating age-neutral reasons for adverse employment actions, as illustrated in *Dalrymple v. George Regional Health System* (2009).

Paulette Dalrymple was an LPN working in the emergency department at George County Hospital. She also worked at Stone County Hospital. Dalrymple applied for FMLA leave in June of 2006 to take care of her spouse. George County Hospital granted her request for FMLA leave, as well as her request to apply the FMLA leave to March and April 2006 absences. She was scheduled to work the first weekends in May and June of 2006, but called in on those days, ostensibly to take care of her spouse. The hospital also permitted her to take FMLA leave for those absences. The hospital policy required that missed weekends be made up, which Dalrymple refused to do. The hospital administrator discovered that she had worked at Stone County Hospital on the May and June weekends she had taken as FMLA leave from George County. She was subsequently terminated for insubordination, falsifying documents, dishonesty, and refusing to make up missed weekends.

Dalrymple filed a complaint with the EEOC alleging age discrimination in her termination. The EEOC dismissed her complaint, and she appealed. As with most discrimination claims, when there is little or no direct evidence of age discrimination, the plaintiff must establish the elements of a circumstantial case. On appeal, Dalrymple's burden was to show that her age actually played a role in the hospital's decision-making process. She needed to show that at the time she was fired, she was a member of the class protected by the ADEA (individuals of at least 40 years of age), that she was otherwise qualified for the position, that she was terminated by the hospital, and that the hospital subsequently hired someone not in the protected class to fill her position.

The hospital argued that the emergency room now used RNs rather than LPNs. New RN positions had been created, and her position no longer existed to be filled. The Court reasoned that it might be a question of fact whether the job qualifications for RNs and LPNs were roughly equivalent. As such, Dalrymple had established a prima facie case of employment discrimination.

Once the plaintiff establishes a prima facie case, the defendant has the opportunity to articulate legitimate, nondiscriminatory reasons for the termination. George County Hospital stated that the termination was based on Dalrymple's refusal to reschedule her missed weekend shifts, insubordination, and dishonesty in leading the hospital to believe she needed FMLA leave for the time she was working at the other hospital. Having established a legitimate, nondiscriminatory reason for the termination, Dalrymple now had to present evidence that those proffered reasons were pretextual. She was unable to do so. Noting that several of the new-hire RNs were in her protected age class and more credentialed, the Court dismissed the discrimination claim against the hospital.

Dalrymple had also claimed retaliation for having exercised her rights under the FMLA. To succeed in a hostile work environment claim, the plaintiff must demonstrate that he or she has exhausted all administrative remedies. To succeed in a retaliation claim, Dalrymple, as in *Staples v. Parkview Hospital, Inc.* (2009) described previously, needed to demonstrate that the hospital's action was based upon having exercised her FMLA rights. The Court dismissed this claim as well, noting that Dalrymple had violated the hospital's weekend scheduling policy, a legitimate, nondiscriminatory reason for her termination.

Equal Pay Act of 1963

The Equal Pay Act of 1963 is intended to prohibit sex-based wage discrimination. Payment must be at the same rate for jobs requiring the same skill, effort, and responsibility, and that are performed under similar working conditions. Exceptions exist to allow higher payments for seniority, merit systems, production quota systems, or any other factor unrelated to sex. Similarly labor organizations may not "cause or attempt to cause" an employer to violate the prohibition against such discrimination [EPA, 1963, § 206(d)(1-2)]. The EPA has been the source of litigation when employers have paid PAs higher wages than NPs, as illustrated in *Beck-Wilson v. Principi* (2006).

NPs employed by the Cleveland Veterans Affairs Medical Center (VAMC) brought suit alleging that they were paid less than PAs performing jobs of equal skill, effort, and responsibility under similar working conditions. They claimed that the disparity reflected sex discrimination, in that more than 95% of the NPs were female and more than 85% of the PAs were male. When NP Beck-Wilson discovered that the NPs were being paid significantly less than PAs despite performing the same work, she addressed her concerns with the director. Not receiving satisfaction, she filed a complaint with the EEOC alleging EPA violations. The case was dismissed and Beck-Wilson, along with 18 other NPs, filed suit alleging EPA and Title VII violations. The NPs claimed that they were more highly educated and had received more training than PAs, yet were paid up to $10,000 less per year. One employee, both a PA and an NP, chose "not to invoke her greater educational qualifications as an NP because under the existing pay schemes she earns more money working as a PA" (*Beck-Wilson v. Principi*, 2006, p. 358).

The VAMC claimed that compensation rates for NPs and PAs were determined by different statutes. The statutes allowed for special pay scale increases to address recruiting and retention problems, and the VAMC had adopted the special pay scale for PAs, but not for NPs. It claimed that a recruitment and retention issue existed for the PAs, but not for the NPs. The defense was that the pay differences were caused by statutory differences, not sex. The district court dismissed the EPA and Title VII cases despite finding that the NPs had established a prima facie case, because it concluded that the VAMC had established that the wage disparity was a result of a factor other than sex. Seventeen of the plaintiffs appealed the dismissal.

The Sixth Circuit of the United States Court of Appeals noted that claims under the EPA do not require proof of discriminatory intent. In an EPA case, the defendant must respond to a plaintiff's successful establishment of a prima facie case with one of four affirmative defenses. (An affirmative defense is one in which the defendant bears the burden of persuasion.) Because the NPs had established a prima facie case, the

VAMC needed to prove that the pay disparity was due to (a) seniority, (b) merit, (c) production quotas, or (d) any factor other than sex. Unlike other discrimination cases, in which the VAMC would only have to assert a legitimate, nondiscriminatory motive, under the EPA, the VAMC had to prove one of the affirmative defenses.

Also unlike other discrimination cases, the NPs had no burden to prove that the VAMC's reasons were pretextual. The NPs had provided sufficient evidence that the NPs and PAs performed essentially the same work and, in fact, were used interchangeably by VAMC. Indeed, the NPs were more qualified for the higher pay rates, as they possessed greater education and skill, "[E]vidence that the positions being compared are fungible can support a prima facie case (*Beck-Wilson v. Principi*, 2006, p. 360). (*Fungible* positions are those that are fully interchangeable.)

The VAMC argued that complete gender diversity was needed to compare classes, meaning that 100% of the PAs would have to be male and 100% of the NPs would have to be female to satisfy the requirements for an EPA case. It argued that because 15% of the PAs were female and 5% of the NPs were male, the NPs had failed to show an appropriate male comparator. (In a discrimination case, a *comparator* is the person against whom the treatment is seen to be less favorable.) The Sixth Circuit held that complete gender diversity was not required and that the focus was not on job classifications or titles, but upon actual job requirements. "Despite the fact that the VAMC NPs are better educated than their PA counterparts, the PAs earn on average $4,655 per year more than NPs at the VAMC...Thus, under the existing pay scheme, with PAs receiving pay under a special GS (General Scale) pay scale and NPs receiving pay under the standard Nursing Pay Scale, female employees are not being compensated in the same way as their male counterparts" (*Beck-Wilson v. Principi*, 2006, pp. 363–364).

The Sixth Circuit did not accept the VAMC's affirmative defense that the disparity in pay rates was caused by the differing pay scale statutes. Nor did it accept the argument that the higher pay for PAs was necessary because the VAMC had problems recruiting and retaining PAs, but not NPs. The Court noted that the EPA's exception for "other factors not related to sex" did not mean *any* other factor, but meant a factor that was adopted for a legitimate business reason: "[T]he VA's failure to issue a special salary rate for NPs at the Cleveland VAMC while at the same time insisting that the special rate for the PAs must continue results in sexually discriminatory pay differences in violation of the EPA.... A reasonable jury could conclude that the VA's argument that it must continue to pay the predominantly-male PAs on a special pay scale is pretextual" (*Beck-Wilson v. Principi*, 2006, p. 367). Because the NPs successfully established a prima facie case of wage discrimination, and because the VAMC had not persuaded the court of their affirmative defense, the Sixth Circuit reversed the district court's dismissal of both the EPA and Title VII cases.

Civil Rights Act of 1991

In the late 1980s, several high-profile decisions of the USSC were thought to weaken an employee's right to sue employers for discrimination and harassment. Under Title VII, employees did not have the right to a jury trial, nor did they have the ability to be compensated for emotional distress or to recover punitive damages. Employees had to prove that adverse employer actions were motivated by discrimination. They were unable to prevail in a case in which actions of the employer created disparate impact on some employees. Workers working abroad for United States-based companies were not protected by Title VII.

Congress responded to the need for further protection by enacting the Civil Rights Act of 1991 (CRA). Under the Act, employees could now ask for jury trials [CRA, 1991, § 102(c)] and sue for compensatory and punitive damages [CRA, 1991, § 102(b)]. Additionally, an employee could establish discrimination by showing that an employer practice resulted in a disparate impact on the basis of a protected classification such as race, color, religion, sex, or national origin. The employer would have to demonstrate that such practices were required by business necessity (CRA, 1991, § 105). The protections now applied to all workers employed by American companies, regardless of international location (CRA, 1991, § 109).

APNs AS CONTRACTORS

APNs should understand what terms to negotiate and have employment contracts reviewed by an attorney prior to signing, so as to fully understand the potential legal impact of each of the agreement's terms. Collaborative practice agreements with physicians must be consistent with the APN's ethical and licensure obligations. They should be written, signed, and dated agreements, with all parties having their own copies. The need for this is illustrated in a recent Louisiana case. In *Moore v. Talbot* (2009), APN Moore discontinued her employment with a practice group and closed her own clinic to accept a position with Dr. Talbot.

She sold her office supplies and medical equipment to Talbot, and agreed to accept wages of $60 an hour, $10 more than her $50 per hour rate at the prior practice group. On her first day of work and every day thereafter, Moore presented Talbot with a collaborative practice agreement that he did not sign.

After approximately 1 week of work, Talbot informed Moore that he was "going in a different direction" and intended to pay her $30 per hour, rather than the $60 per hour as agreed. Moore made a written demand, but Talbot continued to refuse to pay the remainder of the wages due. Moore filed a breach of contract claim and was awarded penalties, costs and expenses, and attorney's fees. Talbot appealed, claiming that he could not be held responsible for paying her as an NP in the absence of a collaborative practice agreement. In Louisiana, collaborative practice agreements are not required unless the NP engages in diagnosis and prescription. The Court found that the lack of a collaborative practice agreement was irrelevant, as Moore and Talbot had entered an oral employment agreement. Because Talbot was obligated to pay Moore the wages due, the award was upheld.

Contract Basics

Dates: Contracts must have the effective dates of the agreement. They may have specific start and end dates with renewal provisions, or they may be open-ended, stating that the relationship will begin on a certain date and remain in effect until one or both of the parties agree to terminate the relationship. Notice periods may be established for such terminations.

Purpose: The agreement should state that the purpose of the contract is to outline the relationship between the physician(s) and the APN. It should be clear that the physician's authority to delegate medical acts to the APN does not apply to independent nursing acts.

Nature of the relationship: The contract should specifically identify the APN as an employee or as an independent contractor.

Amendments: The contract should only allow for modifications of the agreed-to terms upon approval of both parties. Agreements that permit unilateral changes can be detrimental to the interests of the APN and provide little protection.

Patient population: The agreement should provide a general description of the practice and identify the patient population for whom the APN will be responsible.

Location: The agreement should specify the state or states in which the APN will be practicing with the physician and define geographic restrictions. Practice settings should also be identified (hospital clinic, office, home).

Conflict resolution: The agreement should specify the manner in which contractual disputes are to be resolved and who is responsible for attorney's fees.

Noncompetition clauses: The agreement may contain a clause that restricts the APN from providing some or all services anywhere else within a specified mile radius without the permission of the practice. This is known as a "restrictive covenant." The restriction may be for the term of the agreement and for a specified period of time after its termination. The APN should evaluate this clause to make sure it is reasonable and not overly restrictive. Restrictive covenants, or non-compete clauses, are generally considered to be a restraint on trade. They will be enforced, however, when considered to be reasonable in geography and time, as is illustrated in *Washington County Mem. Hosp. v. Sidebottom* (1999).

APN Sidebottom signed an agreement with Washington County Memorial Hospital. The agreement contained a clause that stated she would not work within a 50-mile radius of the hospital without the hospital's consent during the term of the agreement, and for a period of 1 year after termination of the agreement. She requested permission to work for the Washington County Health Department performing prenatal nursing care. The hospital agreed because it was not providing prenatal services at the time. In granting permission, the hospital reserved its right to withdraw that permission if it did start providing those services. Sidebottom resigned from the hospital and accepted a position with a physician whose office was less than 50 miles from the hospital. The hospital obtained a permanent injunction prohibiting her from practicing within 50 miles of the hospital for a period of 1 year from the time of her resignation.

Sidebottom appealed the injunction, arguing that the hospital was not at risk of losing patients because she was working in a medically underserved area and had agreed not to treat the hospital's patients. The Court noted that the noncompetition clause was clear and unambiguous, and that the hospital had notified her before her last day that it would be enforced. Finding that noncompete clause was reasonably necessary to protect the hospital's interests; the Court ruled that it could be enforced.

Termination clause: Language should be clear that the APN cannot be arbitrarily terminated. Continuation of the contracts may be explicitly contingent upon maintaining licensure in good standing, meeting all continuing education requirements, and otherwise remaining qualified to practice. The contract may be automatically terminated for other specified reasons such as criminal indictments, mental instability, chemical addiction, or physical disability. This is illustrated in a 2003 Louisiana case.

In *Gordon v. Hurlston* (2003), CRNA Gordon entered into a contract with Dr. Hurlston. At the time of entering the contract, Gordon had a temporary permit to practice, with an expiration date of February 15, 2000. He continued to work for Hurlston as a CRNA until submitting his resignation in March of 2001. Two days prior to Gordon's last day of work, Hurlston was notified that Gordon was not licensed to provide CRNA services and that Hurlston could not bill for Gordon's services that had thus far not been billed. He was also notified that he would need to reimburse third parties for the amounts of CRNA services he had been billed during the time in which Gordon was not licensed.

Gordon filed a complaint, claiming that he had been an employee and Hurlston did not pay him for 3 weeks that he worked in March of 2001. Under Louisiana state law, employers were required to pay employees any amounts due for work performed. Hurlston filed a countercomplaint, claiming that he was not liable to Gordon under Louisiana state law because Gordon had been an independent contractor. He alleged that Gordon had breached the part of his contract requiring him to maintain licensure, and sought reimbursement for the CRNA services performed during the period when Gordon was unlicensed.

The trial court analyzed whether Gordon was an employee or an independent contractor, and determined that Hurlston had not had the right to exercise enough supervision and control over Gordon to be considered his employer. (Hurlston did not control the manner in which Gordon provided anesthesia; Gordon had the ability to work for other companies; Hurlston paid Gordon a flat rate without deductions; Gordon had the right to conduct direct billing.) The court concluded that Gordon had been an independent contractor. Because he was not an employee, Hurlston was not bound by the Louisiana law that applied to employee–employer relationships. The court also found that the agreement signed by Gordon and Hurlston specifically identified Gordon's CRNA license as a material term of an independent contractor agreement. The responsibility to maintain his CRNA license was Gordon's, not Hurlston's. The court ruled against Gordon, awarding Hurlston $53,354.55 plus attorney's fees.

On appeal, the appeals court upheld the decision against Gordon and the $53,354.55 award, but reversed the attorney's fees, as the contract had been silent on the payment of legal fees for disputes.

Collaborative Practice Agreements and Nurse Practice Act Considerations

Each state defines the scope of practice for all nursing providers in its Nurse Practice Act (NPA). APNs must study and abide by the scope as defined in whichever state or states they practice. APNs must know specifically what their state requires in collaborative practice agreements, particularly regarding diagnosis and prescription. NPAs may specify protocols for resolving diagnostic or treatment disagreements between APNs and physicians. They may also require the collaborative practice agreements to provide for patient record review.

Collaborative practice agreements should specify that the duties expected of the APN will be in accordance with nursing board requirements. This is particularly critical for diagnostic and prescriptive responsibilities. It is important that the agreement contain language such as:

> The professional responsibilities delegated herein are authorized within the scope of practice of _____ (APN title and specialty) as identified by _____ (name and statutory reference to each state's NPA and other regulations). The physician(s) and the APN agree that the authority to administer and dispense drugs and medications will remain consistent with the APN's skill, competence, and formal education.

Specific language should address legend drugs, controlled substances, durable medical equipment, pharmaceutical samples, and drug research. The agreement should state that the collaborating physician accepts responsibility for the manner in which the practice uses the controlled substance authority of the APN, and that it is consistent with the NPA and any other regulatory requirements. The APN's license and DEA number should be noted in the agreement.

The parameters of practice may be directly detailed in the agreement, or it may reference compliance to protocols, standing orders, or clinical pathways. The amount and manner of physician supervision and consultation should be explicit and reference the physician's review of NP diagnosis, documentation, and treatment plans.

Terms

The contract should specify the method and frequency of compensation in wage rates, salary, hourly rate, compensatory time, bonuses, productivity schedules, and/or profit sharing, as well as overtime, on-call pay, and reimbursement for expenses. The amount of the compensation will be determined by the amount of income the APN is expected to generate, balanced by the overhead costs the practice expects to incur in hiring the APN.

The practice may not withhold taxes from the pay of independent contractors, in which case the APN will be responsible for doing so. Compensation may be tied to performance appraisals, and the time frame for the initial evaluation may be a negotiable term. There should be language regarding who conducts the evaluations and with what frequency. The agreement should address how scheduling is done, and address any off-shift, weekend, or holiday expectations. Hospital admission authority and procedures should be clear. Responsibilities for the supervision of other providers or support staff may also be an expected part of the job description.

Benefits such as health insurance, sick time, disability insurance, vacation, personal days, conference fees, tuition, professional organization membership dues, professional journal subscriptions, and pension or other retirement plans may be standard and inflexible, or they may be negotiable. They may not be provided at all for independent contractors. The practice may also agree to pay for other professional expenses, such as license renewal and DEA application fees. APNs are strongly advised to have their own professional liability insurance and not rely on the employer's policy for protection.

Negotiation Tips

Preparation is essential. The APN should be as familiar with the practice as possible. Knowing the patient population, volume, reputation, and philosophy of the practice will place the APN in a better position to negotiate favorable terms. Journal publications may provide information regarding the clinical and research interests of the physicians. Applicants should know whether the practice has previously hired APNs, or if this will be the first time. Talking with APNs or PAs who previously or currently work with the practice can provide "inside" information that can be useful in the interview.

First impressions are critical. The professional-appearing APN is in a better position to negotiate terms. Dressing conservatively and arriving on time are basic requirements to creating a favorable impression. Firm handshakes and eye contact, as well as confidence and attention, suggest competence. As with any job interview, extra copies of a résumé and personal references may be helpful and make the candidate appear prepared.

Having terms in mind and being able to articulate a rationale to support them will allow the negotiations to proceed more smoothly.

The APN should know which terms are non-negotiable, and for which terms compromise is acceptable. Reviewing the APN job description will provide information as to the practice's expectations of that role. As agreeable as the terms may appear, all contracts should be reviewed by an attorney prior to signing. Many professional organizations provide resources and guidance in contract negotiations.

SUMMARY

APNs who work as employees share many common labor and employment issues with all workers. Unless they are defined as "supervisors," APNs are entitled to protections of the NLRA and the same rights as any worker represented by a collective bargaining unit. Legislation may be necessary to resolve the conflict between "professional" inclusion and "supervisor" exclusion from the NLRA.

APNs who work as independent contractors must negotiate collaborative practice agreements that comply with NPA requirements. As independent contractors, APNs must be aware of their tax obligations and negotiate the terms of employment agreements. APNs who work in triangulated relationships may be either employees or independent contractors.

KEY POINTS

1. APN benefit rights and tax responsibilities differ considerably and are based on worker classification.
2. The distinction between employee and independent contractor is determined by many factors related to control over the APN's practice.
3. Regardless of worker classification, APNs are strongly advised to carry personal professional liability insurance, rather than relying on employer policies.
4. Collaborative practice agreements must be negotiated and carefully reviewed by an attorney prior to signing.
5. APNs in triangulated employment relationships must clarify their status to understand their rights and responsibilities.

REFERENCES

Age Discrimination in Employment Act of 1967 (ADEA), 29 U.S.C. Ch. 14 (1967). Retrieved September 7, 2009, from http://finduslaw.com/age_discrimination_in_ employment_act_of_1967_adea_29_u_s_code_chapter_14

Americans With Disabilities Act of 1990 (ADA), 42 U.S.C. Ch. 126 (1990). Retrieved September 7, 2009, from http://finduslaw.com/americans_with_disabilities_act_of_ 1990_ada_ 42_u_s_code_chapter_126

Americans With Disabilities Act Amendments Act of 2008 (ADA Amendments), PL 110-325 § 3406 (2008). Retrieved September 10, 2009, from http://www.eeoc.gov/ policy/adaaa.html

Barker J., & Carlos, E. (2007, December 1). Supervisors under the NLRA: Oakwood Healthcare one year later. *Labor Law Journal.* Retrieved September 17, 2009, from http://www.allbusiness.com/government/government-bodies-offices-us-federal-gov ernment/8891329-1.html

Civil Rights Act of 1964 (CRA), Title VII, Equal employment opportunities, 42 U.S.C. Ch. 21 (1964). Retrieved September 7, 2009, from http://finduslaw.com/civil_ rights_act_of_1964_cra_title_vii_equal _employment_opportunities_42_us_code_ chapter_21

Civil Rights Act of 1991 (CRA), Pub. L. 102-166 (1991). Retrieved September 14, 2009, from http://www.eeoc.gov/policy/cra91.html

Employment Standards Administration, 29CFR541. *Defining and delimiting the exemptions for executive, administrative, professional, computer, and outside sales employees.* Retrieved September 8, 2009, from http://www.dol.gov/dol/allcfr/ESA/Title_29/ Part_541/toc.htm

Employment Standards Administration, 29CFR541.301. *Learned professionals.* Retrieved September 8, 2009, from http://www.dol.gov/dol/allcfr/ESA/Title_29/Part_ 541/29CFR541.301. htm

Employment Standards Administration, 29CFR541.314. *Exception for physician, lawyers, and teachers.* Retrieved September 8, 2009, from http://www.helmsgreene.com/ UploadedFiles/RCL/830200544351PM.pdf

Equal Pay Act of 1963 (EPA), 29 U.S.C. Ch. 8 § 206(d) (1963). Retrieved September 7, 2009, from http://finduslaw.com/equal_pay_act_of_1963_epa_29_u_s_code_cha pter_8_206_d

Fair Labor Standards Act of 1938 (FLSA), 29 U.S.C. Ch. 8 (1938). Retrieved September 7, 2009, from http://finduslaw.com/fair_labor_standards_act_flsa_29_us_code_cha pter_8

Family and Medical Leave Act of 1993 (FMLA), 29 U.S.C. Ch. 28 (1993). Retrieved September 7, 2009, from http://finduslaw.com/family_and_medical_leave_act_fmla_ 29_us_code_chapter_28

Gittleson, J. (2009, June 25). Register settles suit with carriers. *Orange County Register.* Retrieved September 6, 2009, from http://www.ocregister.com/articles/million-carri ers-callahan-2475 215-register-independen

House Resolution 1644. (2007–2008). *Re-empowerment of skilled and professional employees and construction tradesworkers (RESPECT) Act: To amend the National Labor Relations Act to clarify the definition of "supervisor" for purposes of such act.* Retrieved September 18, 2009, from http://www.govtrack.us/congress/bill.xpd?bill=h110-1644

Internal Revenue Service. (2008). Publication 1779, *Independent contractor or employee.* Retrieved September 4, 2009, from http://www.irs.gov/pub/irs-pdf/p1779.pdf

Internal Revenue Service. (2009). Topic 762, *Independent contractor vs. employee.* Retrieved September 4, 2009, from http://www.irs.gov/taxtopics/tc762.html

Labor Management Relations Act of 1947 (LMRA, also known as Taft-Hartley Act), 29 United States Code, Title 29, Chapter 7, §§ 141–197. Retrieved April 15, 2010, from http://www.law.cornell.edu/uscode29/usc_sup_ol_29_10_7.html

Labor-Management Reporting and Disclosure Act of 1959 (LMRDA/Landrum-Griffin Act), 29 U.S.C. 411 Pub. L. 86-257 73 Stat. 519-546 (1959). Retrieved September 15, 2009, from http://www.dol.gov/esa/olms/regs/statutes/lmrda-act.htm

McLean Hospital Corporation and Massachusetts Nurses Association, 311 NLRB No. 127 (June 30, 1993).

National Labor Relations Act of 1935 (NLRA), 29 U.S.C. § 151-169 [Title 29, Ch. 7, Subchapter II] (1935). Retrieved September 14, 2009, from http://www.nlrb.gov/about_us/overview/national_labor_relations_act.aspx

National Labor Relations Board (NLRB). (1989). *Rules and regulations and statements of procedure, subpart C—Appropriate bargaining units § 103.30*. Retrieved September 16, 2009, from http://www.nlrb.gov/nlrb/legal/manuals/RulesRegs/RulesRegsFull.pdf

Oakwood Care Center, 343 NLRB No. 76 (2004).

Pittsburgh Business Times. (2008, December 6). *FedEx to pay $26.8M in Calif. settlement*. Retrieved September 6, 2009, from http://www.bizjournals.com/pittsburgh/stories/2008/12/01/daily52. html?q=fedex%20settlement%20independent%20contractor

Rehabilitation Act of 1973 (September 26, 1973), Public Law 93–112, 93rd Congress, H.R. 8070. Retrieved april 15, 2010, from http://www.doter.ost.dot.gov/Documents/yer/REHABACT.htm

Schiffer, N. (2005, August). Whither vs. wither: How the NLRA has failed contingent workers. *American Bar Association Annual Meeting Section on Labor and Employment Law*. Retrieved September 17, 2009, from http://www.bna.com/bnabooks/ababna/annual/2005/018.pdf

The New York Presbyterian Hospital and New York State Nurses Association, 354 NLRB No. 5 (April 29, 2009).

Time Warner. (2000, November 17). *Press release: Time Warner settles lawsuit with Department of Labor for $5.5 million*. Retrieved September 6, 2009, from http://www.timewarner.com/corp/newsroom/pr/0,20812,668034,00.html

United States Equal Employment Opportunity Commission. (2009). Employment discrimination. Retrieved September 10, 2009, from http://www.eeoc.gov/types/ada.html

United States Equal Employment Opportunity Commission. (2007). Questions and answers about health care workers and the Americans with Disabilities Act. Retrieved September 10, 2009, from http://www.eeoc.gov/facts/health_care_workers.html

Williams, K. (2004, July 23). Ethics: Ethics and collective bargaining: Calls to action. *Online Journal of Issues in Nursing*. Retrieved September 17, 2009, from http://nursingworld.org/MainMenuCategories/ANAMarketplace/ANAPeriodicals/OJIN/Columns/Ethics/EthicsandCollectiveBargaining.aspx

TABLE OF CASES

American Hospital Assn. v. NLRB, 499 U.S. 606 (1991).

Beck-Wilson v. Principi, 441 F.3d 353 (6th Cir. 2006).

Belt v. EmCare, Inc., 351 F.Supp.2d 625 (E.D.Tex. 2005).

Belt v. EmCare, Inc., 444 F.3d 403 (5th Cir. 2006).

Dalrymple v. George Regional Health System, S.D. Miss. (2009).

DiFiore v. American Airlines, Inc., 454 Mass. 486 (2009).

Fair Oaks Anesthesia Associates, P.C. v. National Labor Relations Board, 975 F.2d 1068 (4th Cir. September 17, 1992).

Gordon v. Hurlston, 854 So.2d 469 (La. App. 3 Cir. 9/10/03).

Hammond v. Cty. of Los Angeles, 160 Cal. App. 4th 1579 (2008).

Hospital General Menonita v. NLRB, 393 F.3d 263 (1st Cir. 2004).

McDonnell Douglas Corp. v. Green, 411 U.S. 792 (USSC 1973).

Moore v. Talbot, 5 So.3d 313 (La. App. 1 Cir. 2/13/09).

NLRB v. Health Care & Retirement Corp., 511 U.S. 571 (USSC, 1994).

NLRB v. Kentucky River Community Care, Inc., 532 U.S. 706 (USSC 2001).

NLRB v. St. Francis Hospital of Lynwood, 601 F.2d 404 (9th Cir. 1979).

Staples v. Parkview Hospital, Inc., No. 01:07-CV-327 (N.D. Ind. Mar. 6, 2009).

Vizcaino v. Microsoft Corp., 290 F.3d 1043 (9th Cir. 2002).

Vizcaino v. US Dist. Court for W.D. of Wa, 173 F.3d 713 (9th Cir. 1999).

Vlahos v. Schroeffel, No. 02-CV-0139 (E.D.N.Y. Mar. 6, 2006).

Washington County Mem. Hosp. v. Sidebottom, 7 S.W.3d 542 (Mo.App.E.D. 1999).

6

Licensure and Regulation

EDITH ANN BROUS

The right to practice a recognized profession is not an absolute or unqualified right.

—Gloria Damgaard

INTRODUCTION

Nursing is a regulated profession at all levels of practice. The state legislatures, through administrative procedure acts known as Nurse Practice Acts (NPAs), empower specialized agencies to oversee nursing education, licensure, and practice. These agencies or boards of nursing (BONs) are responsible for ensuring that those who practice nursing are qualified to do so. Nursing boards are charged with protecting the public from unqualified or unsafe practitioners.

After issuing licenses, BONs continue to monitor compliance to the NPA, and the *right* to practice one's profession can be forfeited when the BON finds that the practitioner poses a danger to the health and safety of the public. In that sense, licensure is considered as much of a *privilege* as it is a *right*. This chapter will provide the APN with an overview of BON structure, the regulatory process, and complaint resolution. Such an understanding is essential to maintaining one's license in good standing.

BACKGROUND

In the early 1900s, NPAs were originally simple registry laws, merely listing trained nurses. They evolved into formal practice acts requiring professional licensure and defining standards for nursing practice. Distinct and quite restrictive scopes of practice were delineated for registered nurses (RNs) and practical nurses. As nursing practice expanded, BONs revised the minimum educational preparation and licensure requirements to reflect nursing's evolving scope of practice. Physician's assistant and nurse practitioner (NP) roles emerged in the 1970s in response to a shortage of primary care physicians (Damgaard, Hohman, & Karpiuk, 2000, p. 2). BONs responded by developing specific regulatory schemes for advanced nursing practice.

Although nursing practice roles had been evolving and expanding for decades, the RN scope of practice was not inclusive of advanced practice roles. Existing nursing regulations did not address educational requirements, prescriptive authority, admission and referral privileges, or billing and insurance recognition. Damgaard and colleagues note that the first certification examination for NPs was not available until 1981 (Damgaard, Hohman, & Karpiuk, p. 3).

Board Structure

Each state or territory has a responsibility to protect the welfare of its citizens. Toward that end, states delegate the authority to regulate and monitor licensed professionals to administrative agencies with the necessary specialized expertise to do so. Nursing boards, therefore, are created by individual state law and remain creatures of the particular state. They may be freestanding agencies, subagencies of other agencies, or hybrid organizations. Although individually structured, a common mission for all BONs is protecting the public by defining nursing practice and monitoring its licensees for safe and ethical practice.

Board members are generally appointed by the governor. Senate advice and consent may be required for the governor's selections. The BON may be required to submit a list of candidates to the governor, and/or nominees may be submitted by nursing organizations. The number of board members, their qualifications, and terms of office are state-specific and outlined in the NPA. The composition generally includes advanced practice nurses (APNs), RNs, licensed practical nurses (LPNs), and lay members of the general public. Board members may be required to be United States citizens and residents of the state or territory in which they are appointed. Some states also require that board members be registered voters.

The NPA may require that the nurses on the board be in active clinical practice with a minimum experience prerequisite. Some NPAs require that the board consist of nursing direct providers, educators, and administrators. Educational requirements may also exist for some or all members. Members may serve staggered terms. Officer elections, the filling of vacancies, compensation, if any, removal of members, conflict of financial interest prohibitions, moral character, and other requirements are specifically determined by the state NPA. The NPA may specify the number of meetings the board must have annually, as well as agenda structure, required committees, and member duties. Individual BONs are constituent members of the National Council of State Boards of Nursing (NCSBN).

Board Authority

BONs are governmental agencies with statutory authority to regulate the licensed professions. As such, they may have police and prosecutorial powers, such as the authority to impose penalties and levy fines, the legal right to obtain medical records (those of patients and of the licensees), subpoena power, and the power to issue injunctions or emergency suspension orders. Although licensees have the right to seek judicial intervention, BON decisions are granted great deference by the courts. To appeal a board decision, the licensee must generally demonstrate that the BON was incorrect in its application of the law, exceeded the scope of its authority, or acted in an arbitrary and capricious manner, as discussed in the text that follows.

In *Corcoran v. Board of Nursing* (2005), the Oregon BON issued an order of emergency suspension when a family nurse practitioner (FNP) was accused of sexual and financial misconduct involving multiple patients. Finding a high probability of recurrent acts of sexual misconduct and boundary violations, the BON believed the FNP posed a serious danger to public health and safety. His license, therefore, was immediately and indefinitely suspended. An investigation was conducted, as well as a hearing by an administrative law judge (ALJ) who issued a proposed order finding that the BON's order of immediate suspension had been unfounded.

The BON found the FNP less credible and the complaining patients more credible than the ALJ had. Similarly, the BON found the prosecution expert opinion testimony more credible than that of the defense, whereas the ALJ placed greater credence in the testimony of the defense expert. Due to differing assessments of FNP and witness credibility, the BON's final order differed from the ALJ's proposed order. The BON issued a final order suspending the FNP's license and certificate for no less than 2 years, during which time the FNP was required to undergo evaluation, treatment, and education. The BON also confirmed the correctness of its original emergency order of indefinite suspension.

The Oregon legislature was concerned about potential conflicts of interest and bias when administrative agencies functioned both as fact-finders and as prosecutors. It had responded to those concerns by enacting legislation requiring agencies to use independent hearing officers. The law only allowed the BON to modify that independent hearing officer's (ALJ's) findings of fact if those findings were not supported by a preponderance of the evidence in the record. The FNP sought judicial intervention, arguing that, among other things, the BON erred in modifying the ALJ's order with regard to the original suspension. The Court reviewed the BON and ALJ findings to make independent findings, and agreed with the BON regarding its findings on all but one of the patients.

Board Function

The functions of a BON are consistent with its mandate to protect the public. The BON has the authority and/or statutory mandate to determine educational curricula and approve nursing programs, evaluate applications for licensure and renewal, maintain records of all licensees, define professional misconduct, investigate complaints, and conduct hearings to determine the need for disciplinary action, and impose disciplinary action on licensees. BONs may conduct criminal background checks on applicants for licensure, and mandate that licensees self-report arrests or criminal convictions.

As administrative agencies, BONS perform quasi-legislative, quasi-executive, and quasi-judicial roles. Rule making and the promulgation and adoption of regulations are legislative functions. It is an executive function to monitor and enforce the rules and to impose penalties. Complaint investigations, conducting of hearings, determinations, and decisions constitute judicial activities.

Administrative procedure acts and other regulatory schemes determine the manner in which these functions are performed. The state legislature may intend that standards and scope of practice changes be accomplished through formal rule making to ensure analysis of the validity and potential impact of the rule on patient health and safety. Such requirements generally are designed to allow public comment by members of the nursing profession.

In response to questions or frequently addressed issues, the BON may issue advisory opinions, position papers, or policy statements. Such opinions may only be considered as guidelines, or they may be considered authoritative with the force of rule or regulation. *Nurses Assn. v. Ohio Bd. of Nursing* (1989) illustrates the distinction. The Ohio BON issued a "Position on Administration of Intravenous Fluids by Licensed Practical Nurses," permitting LPNs to administer intravenous fluids. The Ohio Nurses Association (ONA) asked the BON to rescind the position paper from concerns about allowing LPNs to perform functions exclusively within an RN scope of practice. When the BON refused to do so, the ONA sought judicial intervention to prevent implementation of the position paper. It argued that the BON had promulgated a new rule and had violated its rule-making process in doing so.

The BON argued that the position paper was simply advisory as a professional belief of the BON, and not an enforceable rule, because its language used permissive terms such as "may." Reasoning that the position paper was not a rule, the trial court dismissed the ONA complaint. On appeal, the appellate court held that the position paper was incapable of enforcement by the BON because it was "advisory" and not a rule. The ONA continued its appeal, arguing that the position paper created authority for LPNs to perform procedures not previously allowed under the law. The Supreme Court of Ohio reversed the appellate court, holding that the position paper did constitute a rule, because it expanded the scope of practice for LPNs. It held that the BON was required to comply with the state regulatory code's procedure for adopting rules:

> [W]hen a regulatory body such as the board declares that it will permit those persons it regulates to perform certain procedures, the new standard is inherently "enforced" as soon as it is adopted. Simply because the term "may" is used in the position paper does not make the position paper incapable of enforcement.... [T]he true effect of the position paper is that LPNs are now permitted to perform certain additional aspects of IV therapy without the threat of disciplinary action or other penalty levied by the board. (*Nurses Assn. v. Ohio Bd. of Nursing*, 1989, p. 75)

The Ohio Supreme Court based its decision on the position paper's effect, not on the manner by which the BON characterized it. Because the advisory opinion did not merely interpret an already existing standard, but, in fact, established a new regulation regarding LPN practice, the BON was required to follow the statutory mandates for rule making.

SCOPE OF PRACTICE

BONs may or may not be the exclusive state authority over APNs. Some states regulate APNs through the BON along with separate advisory committees, Joint Practice Committees, the Board of Medicine, other regulatory or licensing bodies, or the public health department (Pearson, 2009). As such, APNs must know not only the scope of their practice as defined in the NPA, but how their practice is defined by other regulatory bodies. Additionally, APNs must be familiar with the scope of practice specific to each state NPA in which they are licensed or apply for licensure, particularly regarding prescriptive privileges. This is exemplified in *Arkansas State Board of Nursing v. Jody Marie Morrison* (2004).

Morrison was a Kansas-licensed APN, where prescriptive authority was part of advanced practice licensure. She applied for licensure in Arkansas, unaware that Arkansas had a separate requirement that APNs have collaborative practice agreements (CPAs) to obtain prescriptive authority. The Arkansas BON received Ms. Morrison's CPA, subsequently followed by a letter from the prospective employer stating that she would not be employed and nullifying the CPA. Morrison was advised that her application was about to expire. She informed the BON that she had been writing prescriptions in Arkansas. The BON wrote her a letter advising her that she did not have prescriptive authority, and directing her to immediately cease prescribing medications. She did cease prescribing medications when told to do so, and admitted that she wrote prescriptions but did not know that she lacked authority to do so.

The Arkansas BON, finding her guilty of unprofessional conduct and of writing prescriptions without proper authority, imposed a $1,000 fine, placed her license on probation for 6 months, and ordered her to complete a course in legal and ethical issues. Conditions of probation included that she present each future employer with a copy of the Board's order, that she and her employer submit quarterly reports concerning her safe practice of nursing, and that she not practice nursing outside the State of Arkansas without the written permission of the Arkansas BON and of the BON in any state in which she sought to practice.

Morrison sought judicial review, alleging that the BON's finding that she was guilty of "unprofessional conduct" was not supported by substantial evidence, because the BON failed to produce evidence as to each element necessary to support such a finding of "unprofessional conduct." The circuit court reversed the BON, finding that the BON's decision was not supported by substantial evidence, that there was no proof as to the accepted standards of nursing practice, and that there was no proof that her failure to obtain prescriptive authority was the result of "conscious disregard for the health and welfare of the public and of the patient under the nurse's care."

The BON appealed the reversal, and the appeals court reasoned that Morrison was not simply charged with writing prescriptions without proper authority, but was also charged with "unprofessional conduct." It held that, to prove unprofessional conduct, the BON needed to prove both that an act or omission fell below the standard of care, and that such act or omission was the result of a "conscious disregard for the health and welfare of the public and of the patient." Because there was no proof that her failure to obtain prescriptive authority fell below the standard of care, or that it was done with conscious intent, the Court upheld the reversal.

Similarly, in *Bransfield v. Meconi* (2007), Bransfield, a Delaware-licensed APN, held prescriptive authority for controlled substances. Her renewal application was received 5 days after it was due and was missing a collaborating physician's signature. Controlled-substance registration in Delaware required physician CPAs. Bransfield failed to notify the Delaware Office of Narcotics and Dangerous Drugs (ONDD), Division of Public Health (DPH), and Department of Health and Social Services (DHSS) that her previous physician CPA had been terminated. The following month, Bransfield submitted another renewal application with an unsigned CPA.

When her renewal application was considered untimely and incomplete, an order was issued denying the application. She was advised that her registration had expired and that she no longer had prescriptive authority. She refused to surrender her controlled-substance registration certificates when told to do so, and continued to prescribe narcotic drugs even after being told that she did not have a current registration. Upon appeal, the order denying her application was upheld.

APNs must also stay within the confines of the patient population for whom they are authorized to treat. This is exemplified in *Slagle v. Wyoming State Bd. of Nursing* (1998). Slagle, a licensed geriatric NP, was working in a county jail when the BON received a complaint from a prisoner. The BON asked Slagle to send information about her adult NP standing, and informed her that her license limited her to the care of geriatric patients. She was not advised that there had been a complaint or that the BON was considering disciplinary action.

Slagle's response included descriptions of her training, course work, and university transcript, and stated her belief that she was licensed to practice with an adult population. The BON called Slagle to advise her that she should obtain a specialty license for adult practice but, again, did not advise her that there was a disciplinary matter pending. Slagle sent in qualification information, and requested that her license cover both geriatrics and adults. The BON did not respond, and, despite dismissing the inmate's complaint, it filed a complaint alleging that Slagle exceeded the scope of her license by treating nongeriatric adult patients. The BON suspended Slagle's license for 1 month and issued a "cease and desist order" directing her to stop treating non-geriatric patients. She was also charged with practicing fraud and deceit in submitting false application information. Slagle sought judicial intervention and continued treating adult patients.

The court reversed the BON's actions on the basis that Slagle had not been accorded due process. Reasoning that Slagle's license was a constitutionally protected property right, it held that the BON could not suspend her license without providing her with due process. She was entitled to an opportunity for a hearing and reasonable notice of the asserted charges and the grounds for disciplinary action. It is noteworthy that the court specifically did not decide the issue of whether an APN was limited to practice within one specialty area. The BON action was reversed solely on constitutional grounds.

To practice in an advanced role, nurses must meet the statutory requirements as set out in the NPA. Failure to do so may lead to disciplinary action being taken against one's nursing license, as in *Morris v. Dept. of Prof. Regulation* (2005). In this case, an RN held herself out as a direct-entry/lay midwife, performing prenatal examinations, assisting in deliveries, and providing postpartum and newborn care for a fee. She was not licensed as a midwife, and the Illinois Department of Professional Regulation (IDPR) issued an order for her to cease and desist the practice of midwifery until she was qualified and licensed to do so. The nurse filed a complaint asking for an administrative review of the cease and desist order. She argued that the BON did not have jurisdiction over her as it did not regulate lay midwives, therefore, the cease and desist order was without authority. The Court upheld the BON's order.

The nurse appealed while the IDPR filed a complaint against her, charging her with providing nursing care for which she was not qualified or licensed. Additionally, she was charged with fraud, deceit, and misrepresentation for using the designation CNM (certified nurse midwife). An expert witness testified that nurses may apply for advanced practice licenses only if they have met the legal requirements and have the specified credentials to do so. The nurse's actions (ordering ultrasounds and laboratory tests, providing prenatal care, conducting newborn and postpartum examinations) constituted the practice of advanced practice nursing, in violation of the NPA. The ALJ recommended that her license be suspended for 30 days, followed by a 2-year probationary period during which time she was to complete an ethics course, report her employment activities, and pay a $1,000 fine. The BON adopted some of the recommendations, but suspended her license indefinitely, but at least for 3 years, and increased the fine to $2,500. She was also not to represent herself as a CNM.

On appeal, the Appellate Court of Illinois noted that the IDPR's factual findings would be set aside only if they were against the weight of the evidence. Questions of law would be reviewed *de novo* (as if they were new). This case presented mixed questions of fact and law, and the IDPR's decision would only be reversed if clearly in error. An administrative agency's decision would not be overturned unless the discipline was unreasonable, arbitrary, or unrelated to the purpose of the statute.

The Illinois NPA allowed an RN to practice as a CNM if the RN had:

- applied in writing to the Department of Professional Regulation
- held a current license to practice in Illinois
- completed the requirements to practice and held national certification as a nurse midwife
- paid the required fee
- successfully completed a formal advanced education program in nurse midwifery
- entered into a written CPA with a physician

The Court noted that the nurse did fall within the NPA, such that the IDPR had jurisdiction to discipline her. She had not complied with these licensing requirements, and, as such, the IDPR did nor err in issuing the cease and desist order. Because she was practicing midwifery when not licensed to practice advanced practice nursing, the IDPR also did not err in suspending her license. As the purpose of the NPA was to "promote the public health, safety and welfare by ensuring that those individuals who engage in the conduct described in the Act are properly trained and licensed," the decision to suspend her license and impose a fine was reasonably related to that purpose (*Morris v. Dept. of Prof. Regulation*, 2005, p. 93). The IDPR had not explained the relevance of requiring her to attend an ethics course, however, so the Court vacated that part of the order. The remainder—the suspension, fine, and order to cease and desist the practice of midwifery—was affirmed.

DELEGATION

APNs must know not only their own scope of practice, but also the scope of practice for anyone whom they delegate. The BON may take disciplinary action against a provider for inappropriate delegation. Moreover, many NPAs define delegation and specifically list improper delegation as a form of professional misconduct. BONs may reference delegation in the NPA, their rules and regulations, the standards of nursing practice, educational curriculum requirements, grounds for discipline, or descriptions of nursing practice. Some BONs may also have published advisory opinions, decision trees, guidelines, or identified tasks that may or may not be delegated.

In delegating tasks to others, APNs must consider themselves as ultimately responsible for those delegation decisions. Consideration must be paid to the authorized scope of practice, job description, experience and skill level, and the particular delegatee's competency and performance level.

The National Council of State Boards of Nursing's "Five Rights of Delegation" may serve as a decision framework for determining to whom what may be delegated: right task (one that is delegable for a specific patient), right circumstances (including considerations of the setting and available resources), right person (delegating the right task to the right person to be performed on the right person), right direction/communication (clear, concise description of the task, including its objective, limits, and expectations), and right supervision/evaluation (appropriate monitoring, evaluation, intervention, as needed, and feedback) (National Council of State Boards of Nursing, 1997). Additionally, the American Nurses Association (ANA) and NCSBN have collaboratively published a joint statement on nursing delegation, which provides principles of delegation, decision trees, and useful information for APNs to consider (American Nurses Association & National Council of State Boards of Nursing, 2006).

Delegating acts or responsibilities to an individual who the APN knows, or has reason to know, lacks the ability or knowledge to perform, or failure to adequately supervise and monitor the performance of individuals to whom the APN has delegated nursing acts or responsibilities, may be deemed professional misconduct and lead to disciplinary action. All licensed health care providers must abide by scope of practice limitations of the individuals to whom they delegate, as illustrated in *Lang v. Dental Quality* (2007).

In this case, a licensed dentist and a licensed dentist/physician performed cosmetic and dental surgery in the practice they jointly owned. A complaint was made to the Department of Health, the Dental Quality Assurance Commission, and the Medical Quality Assurance Commission that they allowed unlicensed employees to start intravenous lines and administer general anesthetics, such as Propofol and Versed. A hearing officer imposed a cease and desist order, along with a fine, after finding that they violated statutes specifically prohibiting unlicensed persons from administering general anesthetics. Aiding or abetting an unlicensed person to practice when a license is required constituted unprofessional misconduct.

On appeal, the court affirmed the sanctions, noting that the regulation prohibited the administration of anesthesia by unlicensed personnel, even when under the direction and supervision of the dentist, "[G]iven the serious risk to the public in having unlicensed persons start IVs and administer anesthetic, the sanctions were conservative and not arbitrary or capricious" (*Lang v. Dental Quality*, 2007, p. 255).

APNs must also confine themselves to functions allowed by the BON, regardless of CPAs or physician directives that seek to exceed the allowable scope of practice. This is illustrated in *Wedgeworth v. Spohn Health* (2008). An unwritten policy permitted nurses to prepare patients for endoscopy in the absence of a physician. Such preparations included sedation and the insertion of a colonoscope up to the patient's cecum. After sedating a patient and inserting the colonoscope on one patient, the nurse learned that the physician would not be present to perform the colonoscopy. The nurse, along with a technician, continued the procedure as instructed by the physician. They removed a polyp and performed the entire colonoscopy without the presence or supervision of the physician.

The employer reassigned the nurse to another department and reported her to the BON. The BON did not take any adverse action against the nurse, and she sued her employer for, *inter alia*, fraud, and negligent misrepresentation. The trial court dismissed all elements of the complaint and the nurse appealed.

In her fraud claim, the nurse asserted that the employer falsely represented to her that "[n]urses and staff could perform any delegated task that the nurses and staff were qualified and comfortable performing" (*Wedgeworth v. Spohn Health*, 2008, p. 9). To prevail on that claim, the nurse needed to demonstrate that:

1. A material representation was made
2. The representation was false
3. When the representation was made, the employer knew it was false or made it recklessly without any knowledge of the truth and as a positive assertion
4. The employer made the representation with the intent that the nurse should act upon it
5. The nurse acted in reliance on the representation
6. The nurse thereby suffered injury

The employer argued that the nurse did not demonstrate that it falsely represented its delegation policy, that it intended to deceive the nurse, or that it knew the alleged representations regarding its policy were false. Additionally, the employer argued that the nurse did not present evidence that she relied on the employer's representation regarding its delegation policy. The appeals court agreed with the trial court that the nurse did not demonstrate the employer's intent to deceive and upheld the dismissal of that claim.

To prevail on her negligent misrepresentation claim, the nurse needed to demonstrate:

1. The representation was made by the employer in the course of business, or in a transaction in which it had a pecuniary interest
2. The employer supplied 'false information' for the guidance of others in the business
3. The employer did not exercise reasonable care or competence in obtaining or communicating the information
4. The nurse suffered pecuniary loss by justifiably relying on the representation

The nurse alleged that the employer misrepresented its delegation policy to her. She produced budget and patient volume information, as well as chief nurse executive testimony that the delegation policy was unclear. In addition to claims that the employer had represented that nurses could perform delegated tasks for which they were qualified and with which they felt comfortable, the nurse presented evidence that the employer had also represented that the physician was ultimately responsible for all delegated tasks.

The appeals court agreed that the employer was aware that physicians were delegating procedures to the nurses without being physically present, and that the delegation policy was not clarified until after the incident. The court also agreed that she had suffered a financial loss during the time in which she was being investigated by the BON. Finding that the nurse had demonstrated all elements of her negligent misrepresentation claim, it reversed the dismissal of that claim.

LICENSURE

APNs must be authorized to practice in advanced roles. BONs may require completion of an accredited advanced practice educational program with a minimum number of clinical hours, along with a pharmacotherapeutics course, good moral character, recent clinical experience, verification of a course in state and federal laws related to prescriptions and recordkeeping, and successful completion of a national certification examination. The APN may also be required to submit verification of practice protocols or CPAs before being permitted to practice. Physician involvement may be required for some aspects of practice. APNs may be required to demonstrate continued competence and attend continuing education.

NPAs define the functions APNs may perform that would otherwise exceed the scope of nursing practice. The additional skills and advanced education of an APN may permit diagnosis and primary health management. The scope of practice may be limited to a particular NP certification and/or patient category (National Council of State Boards of Nursing, 2008). Licensure in one jurisdiction does not permit a provider to practice in another without first obtaining licensure in that state, as well. Indeed, practicing without a license constitutes criminal activity, as illustrated in *Lohmiller v. State* (2008).

Lohmiller was licensed to practice nursing in Georgia. She had previously been placed in the federal witness protection program, but withdrew from the program when it would not offer protection to the man she planned to marry. She subsequently moved to Indiana but, out of fear of being found, did not acquire a license in Indiana. She began working in the health department as a public health nurse, signing her name as "RN, MSN." Her position as a public health nurse required her to be licensed as a nurse. The job description specifically detailed that the position required an Indiana nursing license. She had been repeatedly asked for copies of her license and after 4 years of making excuses, finally admitted that she did not possess an Indiana license.

The state of Indiana charged her with Class C felony counts of forgery and Class B misdemeanor counts of practicing nursing without a license. Lohmiller admitted that she signed her name with "RN, MSN," but that she had never been licensed to practice nursing in Indiana. Upon conviction of 6 counts of forgery and 21 counts of practicing nursing without a license, Lohmiller was sentenced to 4 years imprisonment, 2 years of which were to be served in home detention, and 2 years of which were stayed while on probation. She was also ordered to pay $25,000 in restitution. On appeal, the order to pay restitution was reversed and remanded to the trial court to determine actual damages.

COMPLAINT RESOLUTION

BONs become aware of potential problems through a number of sources. Complaints from patients or their families, reports from employers or coworkers, notification by criminal courts, malpractice data banks, or insurance companies, and public information sources, such as the press, all provide the basis for BON investigations. Although the process and statutory authority is specific to each jurisdiction, BONs generally have a legal obligation to investigate all allegations of professional misconduct or gross negligence. Departures from acceptable moral character standards may also result in investigations, even when not directly related to practice.

Some jurisdictions allow verbal complaints, whereas others require that complaints be put in writing. BONs may accept anonymous complaints, or they may require complainants to identify themselves and provide contact information to the BON. (The complaint and identity of the complainant may then be kept confidential by statute or practice.)

Each NPA addresses acceptable and unacceptable conduct on the part of the licensee. Some provide specific definitions of "professional misconduct" or "unprofessional conduct," whereas others generically address the terms. Common activities that may result in disciplinary action by the BON include:

- dishonesty or deceit in the application process and/or obtaining one's license fraudulently

- permitting an unlicensed person to perform activities requiring licensure or improper delegation/supervision/monitoring of delegatees
- practicing with an expired or inactive license or a license currently suspended
- gross negligence or incompetence
- patient abandonment, neglect, or abuse
- practicing while impaired or the habitual use of alcohol or other substances, habitual intemperance or addiction
- practicing beyond one's authorized scope
- criminal convictions
- acts of gross immorality
- disciplinary actions on one's license taken in other jurisdictions
- violations of settlement agreements or consent orders
- failure to abide by probationary terms or to cooperate with an investigation
- participating in unlawful referrals, kickbacks, or fee-sharing arrangements
- falsifying medical or business records or inaccurate, illegible, or incomplete documentation or failure to maintain adequate records
- violations of local, state, or federal laws, rules, or regulations
- noncompliance in continuing education or clinical competency requirements
- accessing or revealing a patient's personally identifiable health information
- failure to notify the BON of name or address changes
- failure to wear identification badges
- failure to observe acceptable infection control practices
- lack of fitness to practice
- mental incompetence or lack of capacity
- "unprofessional conduct" or "professional misconduct"

The BON may call or send a letter to notify an APN that a complaint has been received. The licensee may then be asked to answer a set of written questions called interrogatories, or to appear for an interview to discuss the allegations. APNs have a right to counsel at all stages of a BON action, and should seek legal advice as soon as they are aware that a complaint has been received by the BON. Careful preparation will guide the APN through the process and may improve the outcome. A personal malpractice insurance policy may offer licensure protection as a benefit, and provide referrals and/or payment for legal services. While clearly conveying the intention to fully cooperate, the licensee must immediately identify that he or she wishes to be represented by an attorney before responding to inquiries. Statements should not be made until obtaining counsel, no matter how informal the conversation appears to be.

Although the primary focus of the interview may be the issues surrounding the complaint, the scope of the investigation is not limited to those matters. The licensee must be prepared to discuss any other concerns the investigator wishes to address and answer all questions posed. A great deal of investigation may have been conducted prior to notifying the licensee that a complaint has been received. The BON may have already reviewed performance appraisals, patient medical records, billing records, criminal background information, employer human resource files, prior disciplinary actions, or other materials. The interview may be recorded or transcribed. The investigator may be a professionally licensed nurse or a lay person.

Resolution at this stage or a decision to take further action will be based upon information obtained in the interview and the investigator's impressions of the APN. The recommendation may be to close the file with no further action and notify the complainant that the matter has been resolved. If resolved at this stage, the APN will also be notified that the matter is closed and no action will be taken. Alternatively, the investigator may refer the matter to a prosecutor for more formal investigation. If further investigation is required, the APN may be asked to an informal settlement conference or directed to attend a formal hearing.

The hearing officer or committee may generate formal reports of its findings and recommendations, which may then be considered by other committees before reaching final conclusions. The process may be lengthy and take place over months, or even years. The APN will be advised of the BON's final findings and approval for recommended actions or of a settlement agreement. Potential outcomes include:

- closure of the file with no further action and no findings of misconduct
- censure or reprimand
- corrective or remedial action, such as education or community service
- the imposition of fines or civil monetary penalties
- probation with supervision, periodic employer reports, and/or practice restrictions

■ suspension for an actual period of time, or stayed suspensions during which time the APN may practice on probationary terms

■ acceptance of a surrender of the license, in which the APN voluntarily agrees to return all licenses and cease practice (some jurisdictions may have mechanisms for relinquishing the license that differs from surrender, in that it is not done as part of a disciplinary action or sanction)

■ annulling a license that the BON finds to have been falsely or improperly obtained

■ revocation in which the license is permanently removed, and the APN is forbidden to practice or hold himself/herself out as a nurse or APN

Alternatives to discipline programs may be available to APNs with chemical dependency. The licensee may be required to surrender his or her license and enter a professional assistance plan. Upon entering an approved treatment program, the APN will then be supervised and may be required to demonstrate sobriety and submit to random drug testing for a designated period of time prior to having his or her license restored. Upon return to practice, the APN will be closely monitored for compliance to probationary terms such as worksite supervision, employer reports, continued random drug testing, and practice restrictions. Upon successful completion of probation, the license may be fully restored. These alternatives to discipline plans are generally restricted to providers who have not injured patients and who remain compliant with the treatment program rules.

Licensees must present consistent information to the board. Discrepancies between what is said at the interview and investigation stages cannot differ from what is uncovered at a hearing, as illustrated in a Wyoming chiropractic case, *In The Disciplinary Matter of Greene* (2009). Several patients filed complaints that the chiropractor made sexual advances during treatments. The Wyoming Board of Chiropractic Examiners found the chiropractor guilty of ethical violations of the state Chiropractic Practice Act, and suspended his license indefinitely with specific conditions laid out for reinstatement. The chiropractor appealed and the district court affirmed the board action.

The chiropractor appealed to the Supreme Court of Wyoming, arguing that the board had abused its discretion, that the order suspending his licensed was arbitrary and capricious, that there were evidentiary errors, and that the decision was not supported by substantial evidence. Specifically, he claimed that the board had not admitted evidence of the mental health of one of the complainants, that he had not received notice of evidence and issues the board considered, that the board permitted a non-complaining witness to testify, that the board rejected his expert witness, that the board considered evidence that was too remote to be relevant, and that his due-process rights were violated when the board accessed and used his proposed expert witness's professional licensing records.

The court noted that, "[A]dministrative hearings are governed by [the state Administrative Procedure Act] and administrative agencies acting in a judicial or quasi judicial capacity are not bound by the rules of evidence that govern trials by courts or juries" (*In The Disciplinary Matter of Greene*, 2009, p. 10). It would only overrule the board's decisions regarding the admissibility of evidence if the board abused its discretion. The standard for admissibility of evidence in administrative hearings was:

> [I]*rrelevant, immaterial or unduly repetitious evidence shall be* excluded and no sanction shall be imposed or order issued except upon consideration of the whole record or such portion thereof as may be cited by any party and unless supported by *the type of evidence commonly relied upon by reasonably prudent men in the conduct of their serious affairs*. (*In The Disiplinary Matter of Greene*, p. 11, citing Wyoming Statues, Title, 16, Chapter 2, Section 108)

Although it would review an agency's conclusions of law *de novo*, the Court would affirm those conclusions when they were in accordance with the law. To find that the board's suspension order was arbitrary and capricious, the suspension would need to prejudice the chiropractor's rights. This would entail refusing to admit clearly admissible testimony or failing to make appropriate findings of fact or conclusions of law.

The Court found that the board had not erred in refusing to admit as evidence the mental health records of one of the complainants. Nor did it find any statutory requirement that witnesses file complaints in order to testify. If such a witness was able to provide information relevant to the allegations, the board was permitted to admit her testimony. The board also did not err in admitting evidence of remote acts, because the decision to admit or exclude such testimony was within the board's discretion. There was, therefore, no abuse of discretion.

Administrative Procedure Acts generally require that boards maintain confidentiality of files and information on its licensees, with the exception of licensing or certification decisions. The Court held that the board's decision to exclude the testimony of the chiropractor's proposed expert witness was not a violation of the chiropractor's due-process rights, although it did express concern that the board had used the proposed expert's confidential information in the absence of authorization or release. In Wyoming, the board was obligated to obtain notarized written consent or a court order. Having failed to do so, the prosecutor should not have had access to the records. This represented a failure of the board to follow its own rules. Although the confidential information was obtained, it was not used in the proceedings. The Court, therefore, found that there was no violation of the chiropractor's due-process rights.

The Court also found that the board had provided adequate notice to the chiropractor of the allegations and that it intended to take disciplinary action. In considering the claim that the board's decision was not supported by substantial evidence, the Court noted that the standard was whether clear and convincing evidence was presented, "whether the kind of proof was presented which would persuade a trier of fact that the truth of the contention was highly probable" (*In The Disciplinary Matter of Greene*, 2009, p. 15). The Court held that clear and convincing evidence had been presented to persuade the board of the chiropractor's violation of board rules and ethical standards.

The board had found that the chiropractor's statements during the investigation contradicted those of his hearing testimony. Additionally, his testimony on direct examination differed from his testimony on cross-examination. His statements were not supported by the documentation in his patient's charts. This was sufficient to convince the board that the chiropractor had not met his ethical obligations to his patients or to the profession. The Court affirmed the board's suspension of his license.

PROFESSIONAL MISCONDUCT/UNPROFESSIONAL CONDUCT

Because the right to practice one's profession is a valuable property right, the state can only exclude a nurse from practice after providing due process. This generally requires notice of a hearing and the opportunity to be heard and defend one's case. Additionally, the licensee must have adequate notice and fair warning of what constitutes conduct that may be subject to disciplinary action. The terms "unprofessional conduct" or "professional misconduct" may appear to provide the licensee with little guidance in this regard. Actual patient harm is not necessary for an APN to be charged with professional misconduct or unprofessional conduct. In some cases, a court may hold that the NPA or the BON's rules and regulations are *void-for-vagueness*, such as in *Tuma v. Board of Nursing* (1979).

In this case, a clinical instructor requested to be assigned to a patient receiving chemotherapy. She then had a discussion with the patient and her family about alternative treatments with natural products. The physician ordered the chemotherapy discontinued when the patient changed her mind, and then resumed it when the patient and her family decided to continue the chemotherapy. The hospital complained to the BON that the nurse had interfered with the physician–patient relationship. When a hearing officer found the nurse guilty of unprofessional conduct, the Idaho BON suspended her license for 6 months.

The nurse appealed her suspension to the court, arguing that because the NPA did not specifically define unprofessional conduct, she was not adequately warned that such conduct would subject her to disciplinary action. The *void-for-vagueness* doctrine, as it is called, is a proposition that to be enforceable, an administrative rule must provide definite standards by which both the licensee and the agency may be guided. The BON argued that, as a professional licensing agency composed of nursing experts, the BON was able use its own expertise in determining standards. The disciplinary action was upheld, and she appealed to the Supreme Court of Idaho.

The Supreme Court considered whether her due-process rights were satisfied when the statute authorized suspension of her license for "unprofessional conduct," but did not specifically define that term. The Court noted that from enactment of the first NPA in 1951 until the time of the case, the BON had statutory authority to adopt and revise rules and regulations, yet had never further defined unprofessional conduct. The nurse was disciplined for interference with the doctor–patient relationship, conduct that the BON had not declared unprofessional. A BON regulation must be sufficiently clear and "definite enough to provide a standard of conduct for those whose activities are prescribed as well as a standard by which the agencies called upon to apply it can ascertain compliance therewith" (*Tuma v. Board of Nursing*, p. 80).

The Court noted that nothing in the statutory definition of "unprofessional conduct" would have warned the nurse that discussion with a patient as to alternative therapies would result in licensure suspension, nor did the BON rules prohibit such conduct. For the BON to use its expertise alone in determining whether or not the nurse's action constituted "unprofessional conduct" would violate the nurse's due-process rights. Additionally, it would not produce uniform standards. Moreover, the hearing officer who found her guilty of unprofessional misconduct was not a nurse, therefore not possessed of the expertise that the BON claimed was within its purview. Finding that the BON rules had not provided a clear definition of unprofessional conduct, the Court reversed the BON order suspending the nurse's license.

Unlike Tuma, courts may determine that even vague language provides licensees with adequate notice of what constitutes unacceptable standards of practice, as in *Stephens v. Pennsylvania St. Bd. of Nursing* (1995). In this case, an LPN was found guilty of unprofessional conduct in permitting a nursing attendant to self-administer a controlled substance and to mistreat a nursing home patient. The nurse argued that the NPA was unconstitutionally vague, in that the term "unprofessional conduct" did not provide a standard by which her conduct could be measured. The hearing officer ruled that she was not subject to disciplinary action and ordered that the charges be dismissed.

The BON reversed this decision, and ordered that she be formally reprimanded and assessed a fine. The nurse sought judicial intervention, and on appeal, the court reasoned that the language would not be unconstitutionally vague unless it failed to "convey sufficiently definite warning as to proscribed conduct when measured against common understanding and practices" (*Stephens v. Pennsylvania St. Bd. of Nursing*, 1995, p. 74). Although the term "unprofessional conduct" did not provide a precise standard, the language could be interpreted within the context of common knowledge and understanding of the members of the nursing profession. The standards of nursing practice required that an LPN protect a patient from abuse and that the nurse not knowingly assist another person to violate a law or BON regulation. These standards were sufficient to provide warning to the licensee that violations may constitute professional misconduct. As such, the court affirmed the order of the BON.

APPEALING BOARD OF NURSING DECISIONS

Because disciplinary action may deprive a person of a benefit or entitlement of licensure, the BON must follow its own rules and regulations in conducting proceedings. A departure from such rules and regulations may create due-process violations for the licensee. APNs who think their due-process rights have been violated, or who believe the BON decision is in error, may seek judicial intervention. Courts, however, are reluctant to overturn licensing board decisions, holding that the BON specialized expertise entitles their decisions to great discretion. Generally, courts will not review cases *de novo*, but will defer to the BON's findings of fact and consider only questions of law.

In seeking judicial intervention to appeal a BON decision, the licensee must understand that a court will only overturn an administrative agency action under narrow circumstances. Generally, those circumstances are limited to:

- the BON did not follow its own procedures and the failure to do so prejudiced the licensee's ability to prepare or present a defense
- the BON decision was arbitrary and capricious
- the BON exceeded the scope of its authority
- the licensee was not granted sufficient due process or the BON committed constitutional violations
- the BON did not resolve the complaint in a timely manner
- the BON's findings of fact were unsupported by substantial evidence (substantial evidence is relevant evidence a reasonable mind might accept as adequate to support a conclusion)
- the BON committed errors of law
- the licensee was not provided adequate notice of a hearing or the opportunity to be heard

In *Arcand v. Brd. of Reg. in Nursing* (2007), the Massachusetts BON imposed a reprimand on an RN. The conduct for which she was charged occurred in 1999, the hearing took place in 2004, and the final decision was rendered in 2006. Between the time of the conduct and the time of the final decision, new regulations came into effect. A reprimand, under the old regulations, did not constitute a form of disciplinary action for purposes of application for licensure in another jurisdiction. The new regulations did require nurses to report reprimands when applying for licensure in other states. The nurse claimed she was prejudiced by the 7-year period it took the BON to process the misconduct claim. Had the BON resolved the complaint in a timely fashion, the old regulations would have been in effect at the time of the final decision. She requested that the old regulations apply, such that she would not need to report the reprimand when applying for licensure in another state.

The Massachusetts Superior Court noted that the 7-year period to process the matter constituted BON incompetence, and violated the state requirement for a just and speedy determination of every procedure. Such delay constituted unlawful and abusive procedures and was very prejudicial to the licensee. Finding the BON action unconscionable and intolerable, the court dismissed the complaint against the nurse with prejudice. (*With prejudice* means the BON was barred from bringing the complaint again.)

In *Devers-Scott v. Office of Prof. Regulation* (2007), after conducting a lengthy hearing, an administrative law officer (ALO) found that a nurse midwife had committed multiple acts of unprofessional conduct and failure to practice competently with three different patients. His ruling 3 months later permanently revoked her license to practice midwifery. She appealed to the superior court and the BON action was affirmed. On further appeal, the Supreme Court of Vermont noted that it would affirm the ALO's factual findings whenever they were supported by substantial evidence. Additionally, it would affirm the ALO's conclusions of law whenever they were "rationally derived from the findings and based on a correct interpretation of the law" (*Devers-Scott v. Office of Prof. Regulation*, 2007, p. 7).

In this case, the court was willing to review the matter *de novo*, as the nonexpert ALO was not a midwife, and therefore did not have the specialized expertise that would entitle his findings to the court's deference. In doing so, however, it found no error in the ALO's findings or conclusions. Additionally, the court found the sanction of revocation reasonable and upheld it: "[A]lthough we will not defer to sanction determinations by nonexpert ALOs, to the same extent as we do to those imposed by expert boards, even that more searching review reveals no error here…[T]he record not only substantially supports, but virtually compels, the conclusion that Devers-Scott repeatedly engaged in unprofessional conduct and provided substandard care to her patients" (*Devers-Scott v. Office of Prof. Regulation*, 2007, p. 60).

A court may reverse a BON order upon a finding that the evidence against the licensee was insufficient, as in *Elshoff v. North Carolina Bd. of Nursing* (2008). The BON notified a home care nurse that she "may not be safe and competent to practice nursing or [she] may have violated the Nursing Practice Act," based upon actions taken in the patient's home. The nurse had conducted a search of the patient's home upon discovering a missing controlled substance. The BON stated that such actions threatened and intimidated the patient. She was given the option of an administrative hearing, a settlement conference, or to be issued a letter of reprimand, as well as probation. After a hearing, the BON issued a letter of reprimand and ordered her to complete an ethical/legal decision-making course. The nurse appealed and the superior court affirmed the BON decision.

Upon further appeal, the North Carolina Court of Appeals considered whether there was substantial evidence to justify the BON's decision. The BON's position was that the nurse's actions had a harassing or intimidating effect on the patient. The BON also argued that the court should uphold its final decision and order by granting deference to its interpretation of its own rules. North Carolina law allowed the BON to discipline licensees whenever satisfied that the licensee had *willfully* violated any of its rules. The Court reasoned, therefore, that the complaint should be dismissed unless the BON could produce evidence that the nurse had *willfully* committed actions for the purpose of harassing or intimidating the patient. The patient's distress represented a subjective effect and was not the test of the nurse's willfulness. The Court found the BON had not presented evidence that her searching for the medication was for the purpose of harassing or intimidating the patient. For that reason, it reversed the trial court's affirmation of the board action and remanded the matter back to that court for the complaint to be dismissed.

Administrative agencies must conduct hearings and make determinations consistent with their statutory authority, but licensees must raise objections during the process, or they may waive their right to do so, as illustrated in the Vermont dental case, *In Re Lakatos* (2007). In this case, a dentist was charged with unprofessional conduct. The Vermont Board of Dental Examiners notified the dentist that it would conduct an evidentiary hearing before a committee composed of three members, a dentist, a dental hygienist, and a lay person. A presiding officer would then propose a decision to the board. The dentist was advised that he would have an opportunity to file exceptions and present briefs and arguments regarding the proposed decision.

The hearing committee concluded that the dentist committed unprofessional practice and issued a decision. The board reached the same conclusion as the hearing committee, but declined to adopt its proposed decision regarding sanctions. It suspended the dentist from practice for 6 months, imposed conditions for reinstatement, and then required that his practice be supervised by a licensed dentist for 2 years.

On appeal, the trial court concluded that the hearing committee procedure used by the board had not been authorized by state law and violated the dentist's due-process rights. It noted that the state law did not specifically authorize the board to appoint a hearing officer to conduct a hearing that would otherwise be heard by the board, as was done in this case. The court also found that due process required the board to be personally present at the hearing when the decision rested materially on credibility determinations. In such a case, it was essential that the board personally observe the witnesses. It reversed the board's decision and remanded for a new hearing.

The board appealed, and the Supreme Court of Vermont noted that, although not specifically authorized by state law, the hearing committee procedure used by the board was also not specifically prohibited by law either. The dentist had not challenged the procedure and had not raised objections to it during the process. This amounted to a waiver of any objection. Additionally, the Court found that the board's decision was based upon objective evidence using its expertise. Demeanor and credibility assessments were not material, and thus did not require the physical presence of the board.

Although finding that the dentist had waived any challenge to the hearing process, it did find that the board departed from the hearing process when rejecting the committee's proposed decision. By issuing its own decision without affording the dentist the opportunity to comment and object, the board violated the dentist's due-process rights. As such, the Court remanded to the board so the dentist could object to the decision.

LEGAL DISABILITY

In some jurisdictions, providers who have lost their licenses or have practice limitations imposed on them as a result of addiction may be eligible for disability. In *Berry v. The Paul Revere Life Ins. Co.* (2009), an anesthesiologist became addicted to prescription drugs. He was accused of practicing under the influence of Demerol during a tubal ligation, resulting in a patient being rendered in a permanent vegetative state. An investigation revealed that the anesthesiologist had diverted narcotics from patients in five cases. His medical licenses in three states were suspended. The Louisiana State Board of Medical Examiners Consent Order specifically prohibited Dr. Berry from practicing in the field of anesthesiology or pain management, as well as from prescribing, dispensing, or administering controlled substances. The restrictions were to be in place for the remainder of his medical career.

Dr. Berry filed a disability claim from which he received benefits for 2 1/2 years. Having been drug-free and in continuous rehabilitation, the insurance company deemed him disabled no longer and discontinued his benefits. He brought an action against the insurance company, claiming that his addiction rendered him permanently disabled. Returning to the practice of anesthesiology would require him to risk relapse by exposing him to controlled substances. The court agreed with the insurance company that Dr. Berry's risk of relapse did not constitute present disability and dismissed the claim.

On appeal, the court reasoned that the prohibitions from practicing anesthesiology rendered Dr. Berry legally totally disabled. The policy did not distinguish between mental and physical disabilities, and did not treat the risk of relapse from physical and mental disabilities differently. As such, the policy did not exclude the risk of relapse for drug addiction. The court, therefore, found that Dr. Berry's claim against the insurance company should not have been dismissed and sent the matter back to the trial court.

Other courts may reason differently, as in *Stanford v. Cont. Cas. Co.* (2008). When a certified registered nurse anesthetist (CRNA) became addicted to Fentanyl, the BON restricted his license, forbidding him from working as a CRNA or having access to narcotics. He received disability benefits and returned to work after completing an addiction program, but relapsed and applied again for long-term disability benefits. The insurer determined that he was not suffering from an impairment that prevented him from working as an anesthetist and terminated his benefits, asserting that the policy did not cover the "potential risk of relapse." The court dismissed CRNA Stanford's suit against the insurer.

On appeal, the court reasoned that because the CRNA was not physically or mentally disabled, he was able to perform another job that did not require administering Fentanyl. In finding the insurance company position to be reasonable, it upheld the dismissal of the CRNA's case.

COLLATERAL IMPLICATIONS

Discipline on one's nursing license, whether as an LPN, an RN, or an APN, may lead to other problems for one's practice and damage a career. The provider may be excluded from participation in the state Medicaid program and/or the federal Medicare program because the BON has imposed disciplinary action. One does not have to be a direct biller for this to be an issue. Being placed on the exclusion list prohibits the licensee from being employed by any employer who receives those funds, severely limiting employment options.

Disciplinary sanctions may be published on the Internet and remain permanently available to the general public, even long after the matter has been resolved and full privileges restored. Reputation damage is very difficult to overcome, and may remain with the licensee for the remainder of his or her career. Prospective employers conducting licensure verification may be deterred from hiring an APN on the basis of prior disciplinary action by the BON, even when that APN is currently in good standing.

Adverse actions taken against a health care professional's license are reported to data banks such as the National Practitioner Data Bank (NPDB) and the Healthcare Integrity and Protection Data Bank (HIPDB). Although access to the information in these data banks is not available to the general public, they may be accessed by prospective employers and hinder one's ability to be hired, enter into collaborative practice arrangement with physicians, or obtain privileges.

Should the event that gave rise to the nursing board complaint also result in a medical malpractice lawsuit, BON findings and final decisions or orders may be discoverable to the plaintiff's counsel and admissible as evidence against the APN. Similarly, should the event also result in a criminal investigation, BON actions against the licensee may be available to assist the prosecutor's case against the APN.

The emotional and psychological impact on the licensee of an adverse BON action cannot be overstated. The process may be enormously stressful, even when resulting in a favorable outcome. Separation from practice due to suspension, surrender, or revocation of a license may make it difficult, or even impossible, to ever return to practice. APNs may require professional support to cope with what can amount to a traumatic experience.

SUMMARY

APNs are responsible for understanding the licensure requirements of the state practice acts for each jurisdiction in which they practice. The purpose of professional practice regulation is protection of the safety and welfare of the public. BONs are charged with establishing nursing standards, responding to complaints, and imposing disciplinary action, when warranted, to protect the public from unsafe or unethical licensees. Although clinical practice is one area of concern, BONs also address issues of moral character. Courts generally view administrative agencies as experts whose findings of fact and final decisions are to be granted great discretion and deference. Overturning a BON disciplinary action requires that the appealing licensee demonstrate the few circumstances under which the court may do so.

APNs must view licensure as a *privilege*, more than as a *right*, and have a broad perspective of what is required by their NPA to maintain one's license in good standing. Typically, employer malpractice policies on licensees do not provide coverage for the defense of licensure actions. Personal malpractice policies may provide licensure protection as a benefit. Licensure investigations, hearings, and settlement negotiations can be financially draining, and such insurance policies may assist the APN in affording legal services for the proceedings. Attorneys experienced in administrative agency proceedings may assist the APN in obtaining more favorable outcomes, as well as providing support and guidance through an extremely stressful experience.

KEY POINTS

1. APNs must be familiar with the NPA of each state in which they practice, and abide by the stated clinical practice standards, scope of practice limitations, and moral character requirements of those acts.
2. Nursing boards are not in place to serve as advocates for licensees or the nursing profession, but to safeguard the public by ensuring that those licensed to practice are qualified to do so.
3. Complaint resolution may be a time-consuming and complicated process, and final determinations or sanctions by the BON are likely to be affirmed by the courts to which the licensees appeal.
4. APNs who suspect or are informed that a complaint has been filed with their licensing board should immediately seek counsel experienced in administrative law, and not attempt to negotiate the process without legal representation.
5. Personal professional liability insurance policies may defray some of the costs of the legal expenses incurred for representation during licensure proceedings.

REFERENCES

American Nurses Association & National Council of State Boards of Nursing. (2006). *Joint statement on delegation*. Retrieved December 7, 2009, from https://www.ncsbn. org/Joint_statement.pdf

Damgaard, G., Hohman, M., & Karpiuk, K. (2000). *History of nursing regulation*. Retrieved November 3, 2009, from http://doh.sd.gov/boards/nursing/Documents/ WhitePaperHistory2000.pdf

National Council of State Boards of Nursing. (1997). *The five rights of delegation*. Retrieved November 17, 2009, from https://www.ncsbn.org/Five_Rights_of_Dele gation_NEW.pdf

National Council of State Boards of Nursing. (2008). *Consensus model for APRN regulation: Licensure, accreditation, certification & education.* Retrieved November 3, 2009, from https://www.ncsbn.org/7_23_08_Consensue_APRN_Final.pdf

Pearson, L. (2009). The Pearson report: The annual state-by-state national overview of nurse practitioner legislation and healthcare issues. *American Journal for Nurse Practitioners, 13*(2). Retrieved November 2, 2009, from http://www.webnp.net/downloads/pearson_report09/ajnp_pearson09.pdf

TABLE OF CASES

Ar. State Board of Nursing v. Morrison, 88, Ark. App. 2002 (2004).

Arcand v. Brd. of Reg. in Nursing, No. 20063530 (Ma. Super. Jun. 28, 2007).

Berry v. The Paul Revere Life Ins. Co., 2008-0945 (La. App. 1 Cir. 7/9/09).

Bransfield v. Meconi, 06A-04-003 (JTV) (Del. Super. 9-28-2007).

Corcoran v. Board of Nursing, 197 Or. App. 517 (2005).

Devers-Scott v. Office of Prof. Regulation, 918 A.2d 230 (Vt. 2007).

Elshoff v. North Carolina Bd. of Nursing, 658 S.E.2d 65 (N.C. App. 3-18-2008).

In re Lakatos, 939 A.2d 510 (Vt. 2007).

In the Disciplinary Matter of Greene, 2009 WY 42.

Lang v. Dental Quality, 138 Wn. App. 235 (2007).

Lohmiller v. State, 884 N.E.2d 903 (Ind.App. 2008).

Morris v. Dept. of Prof. Regulation, 356 Ill. App.3d 83 (2005).

Nurses Assn. v. Ohio Bd. of Nursing, 44 Ohio St.3d 73 (1989).

Slagle v. Wyoming State Bd. of Nursing, 954 P.2d 979 (Wyo. 1998).

Stanford v. Cont. Cas. Co., 514 F.3d 354 (4th Cir. 2008).

Stephens v. Pennsylvania St. Bd. of Nursing, 657 A.2d 71 (Pa. Commw. 1995).

Tuma v. Board of Nursing, 100 Idaho 74 (1979).

Wedgeworth v. Spohn Health, 13-05-446-Cv (Tex. App. [13th Dist.] 4-10-2008).

7

Nursing and Law Pedagogy for Advanced Practice Nurses

DIANE KJERVIK

Evolving and expanding our environmental metaparadigm will encourage us to practice, educate, and do research in the global arena in order to affect the widespread major health problems of our present day.

—D. Kleffel

Legal decisions are complex, and vary according to the state in which the advanced practice nurse (APN) practices. By 2015, APNs are to be prepared for advanced practice by obtaining a doctorate (AACN, 2009). For APNs to become leaders of policy development, which is the expectation of the Doctors of Nursing Practice (DNPs) degree, these APNs will need to be well versed in the law, which includes an understanding of health care policy supported by ethical foundations. The American Association of Nurse Attorneys (TAANA) (Brooke et al., 2003) offers a model curriculum for nursing programs that includes topical areas that must be covered, including, for instance, the U.S. jurisprudential system, administrative law, the nurse–patient relationship, negligence and malpractice, informed consent, intentional torts, documentation, patients' rights, liability insurance, adversarial system, and alternative dispute resolution. Several nursing theorists place law or policy considerations within the concept of environment. This chapter reviews nursing theory that incorporates legal or policy components, teaching strategies to build the APN's understanding of law, and research methods to explore and discover connections between law and advanced practice nursing.

LAW AND NURSING THEORY

In the formative years of nursing, Florence Nighingale posed her view of the importance of environment. Her approach included care of the physical environment surrounding the individual patient to assist the patient to recover; care of the community in which the patient lived to promote the common good; and the use of political skills to change social, economic, and political conditions (Kleffel, 2006). Like Nightingale, Lillian Wald addressed environmental influences that she believed affected health, and used her political influence to bring about changes in the cultural, social, physical, and economic landscape to improve health and reduce poverty (Kleffel, 2006). However, the view of environment constricted when hospitals became the primary place of employment in the early 1930s. As Kleffel (2006) points out, in the hospital setting, nurses lost much of their autonomy, and the immediate surroundings of the patient in the hospital became the greatest concern. Thus, environment was seen as external to the patient and the illness. Public health nursing faded into the background of nursing at this time, as did the concept of environment, until it was revived in the 1970s.

In the 1970s, Martha Rodgers and Jacqueline Fawcett's theories included environment as a key component of, rather than external to, health care (Kleffel, 2006). Society underwent a dramatic change in the 1960s as civil rights emerged as a powerful societal commitment to underrepresented minorities and women. Whether this stimulated the view of the centrality of the environment in nursing theories is unknown, but these theories did address, and continued subsequently to accept, the importance of environment. Theorists in the 1980s such as Chopoorian, Butterfield, and others continued the exploration of environment as part of nursing theory, several emphasizing the sociopolitical influence of the environment and its impact on health (Kleffel, 2006). Also, White (2006) critiques Carper's ways of knowing (empirics, esthetics, ethics, and personal) in nursing by adding a fifth way, sociopolitical knowing, which she says is, "essential to an understanding of all the others" (p. 147). This form of knowing includes the context within which the nurse–patient relationship exists and in which the profession of nursing exists. The visibility of those in power is critical to this understanding, and White (2006) suggests that nurses must learn the importance of gatekeepers within political arenas so that their work to change policy becomes visible to the public. Clearly, law is a gatekeeper in the process of bringing about contextual change in nursing environments. However, as Yeo (1997) points out, efforts to develop nursing science have "blinded" the profession to ethics and values inherent in nursing theories (p. 191). Could it be that legal phenomena have also been invisible to nursing theorists?

As global realities emerged on the political scene, nursing theorists, such as Sister Calista Roy and Jean Watson, espoused the integrative unity of humans with the world, and other theorists advocated that nurses should take action to change the environment to improve health (Kleffel, 2006). When law as a sociopolitical influence affects health outcomes, nurses take action to change those policies. The study of the impact of legal decisions on health is commonly referred to as therapeutic jurisprudence (TJ), a term developed by law professors David Wexler and Bruce Winick in the 1990s to expand the work of the law to examine its broader influence, particularly on mental health (Wexler & Winick, 1996). TJ is a form of policy analysis that studies the process of making policy decisions and the impact these policies have after adoption (Majchrzak, 1984). By embracing legal phenomena as worthy of study in terms of the impact of law on health outcomes, nurses will be able to understand and be in the position to influence change in law by using evidence from scientific investigations, as well as their advocacy skills.

In their educational programs, requirements for sophisticated use of policy expertise by APNs are increasing. The American Academy of Nurse Practitioners' (AANP) *Position Statement on Nurse Practitioner Curriculum* (2007) makes no mention of policy, although the role of advocate is mentioned. Also, two required content domains address management and negotiation of health care delivery systems and cultural competence, which may include policy-level activities, but these are not stated specifically. This statement is addressed to nurse practitioners (NPs) who are educated at MSN and post-MSN levels, with recognition that the requirement of doctoral preparation is on the horizon. When the DNP degree is addressed, policy understanding, development, and advocacy are a major focus of the curriculum.

The American Association of Colleges of Nursing's (AACN) Fact Sheet on the DNP (2009) points out that the current credit expectations of MSN programs are equivalent to required credits in other health professionals' doctoral degrees. Therefore, the AACN believes the required degree for the APN should become the DNP. The Fact Sheet also points out that the DNP should be the terminal practice degree for APNs, much as the PhD is the terminal research degree in nursing. The AACN's *Essentials of Doctoral Education for Advanced Nursing Practice* (2006) identifies health care policy as an essential category of education for APNs. Content regarding leadership must prepare the DNP graduate to be an agent of change "at organizational and policy levels" (p. 10). The graduate is to learn political activism and policy development to "assume a broad leadership role on behalf of the public as well as the nursing profession" (p. 13). In addition, the graduate must have the ability "to engage proactively in the development and implementation of health policy at all levels, including institutional, local, state, regional, federal and international levels" (p. 14). Sophisticated understanding of the law and use of legal research methods will enhance the ability of the DNP to develop, and then change, policy. In fact, the *Essentials* document says specifically, "role preparation for specialty nursing practice, including legal and regulatory issues, is part of every DNP program's curricula" (p. 16).

Faculty who teach in DNP programs may wonder about the form of scholarship that will be recognized in academia. The AACN *Essentials* document (2006) recommends that the form of scholarship best exemplified by DNPs is the scholarship of application, as articulated by Ernest Boyer of the Carnegie Foundation for the Advancement of Teaching (1990). This form of scholarship includes, "the translation of research into practice and the dissemination and integration of new knowledge" (AACN, 2006, p. 11). Products of scholarship include traditional forms such as grants, refereed publications, and peer review of others' work, but also, "practice improvement products such as reports, guidelines, protocols and toolkits" (p. 21).

To assist schools of nursing that offer DNP degrees, the National Organization of Nurse Practitioner Faculties (NONPF, 2005) suggests online curriculum templates for these programs. Two of the templates are for post-MSN programs, and two are for post-BSN programs. The post-MSN templates offer five- or six-semester (2-year) variations, and the post-BSN templates offer nine-semester (3-year) options. The four templates include policy, leadership, and ethics courses, either freestanding, or in combination with one another. Policy leadership in the health care arena is clearly an expectation of the DNP, and as such, these leaders will provide not only excellent patient care, but are well prepared to make major changes in policy that affect health care outcomes.

TEACHING STRATEGIES TO INCORPORATE THE LAW INTO ADVANCED PRACTICE NURSING PROGRAMS

In referring to the incorporation of evidence-based practice into nursing curricula, Pierce (2005) says, "curriculum evolution occurs when a concept is seamless and fully integrated as a value" (p. 239). Although this viewpoint might be true for certain areas of knowledge, such as the use of evidence in practice, integrating law or ethics concepts into several DNP courses might not fit easily, due to the specialized theory and application involved. Instead, free-standing, separate courses taught by knowledgeable faculty might provide more information and guidance about interpretation of the standards and principles involved than integration of this content throughout the curriculum. In fact, the *Model Curriculum of Legal Content in Nursing Education*, published by The American Association of Nurse Attorneys (Brooke et al., 2003), recommends that a separate course taught by nurse attorneys and bioethicists is the ideal way to convey complex legal knowledge to undergraduate and graduate nursing students. Pappas, Clutter, and Maggi (2007) offer a description of a legal seminar for nursing students that includes modules related to the emancipated minor, lawsuits against hospitals, nursing malpractice, supervisory liability, MDs' orders, documentation, and end-of-life issues. They recommend that nurse attorneys provide a valuable role in the course, as they can discuss, "patient examples of how the law applies to various areas in nursing practice" (p. 200). The authors also provide several case examples that faculty can use to discuss law and ethics applications to practice to help students learn principles and decision making involved.

One study of nursing educators and beginning students' views of how to teach nursing codes of ethics in Finland discovered that opinions from faculty and students generally supported integration of ethics content across the curriculum, but some thought that separate courses taught by professionals with expertise in ethics would enhance certain topics (Numminen, Arend, & Leino-Kilpi, 2009). The authors point out that no research has evaluated the realities of integrating ethics codes into nursing curricula, and that, "nurse educators' knowledge of the content and function of the codes and their competence to teach ethics requires exploration, particularly for integrated teaching" (p. 80). Whether the findings of this study would extend to similar findings in doctoral education is worth considering insofar as the doctoral degree, whether research-or practice-focused, requires in-depth understanding of the fields of knowledge that intersect with nursing. Although many nursing faculty are familiar with and use evidence-based practice information, they are not as familiar with ethical tenets, legal research, and findings. In these situations, experts in law and ethics are quite valuable, and can most efficiently teach this information in one course, rather than across many.

Interestingly, the AACN (2006) *Essentials* document that describes doctoral education for advanced practice mandates that certain courses be taught separately for three areas of content: "advanced health/physical assessment, advanced physiology/pathophysiology, and advanced pharmacology" (p. 18). AACN justifies this mandate by saying that it, "ensures sufficient depth and focus" (p. 18). However, other content areas also require depth and focus, as well as well-prepared faculty, to succeed in conveying the information and application. There are two foci for DNPs recommended by AACN (2006), one for APNs and the other for systems or policy specialties. For those with public policy goals, a separate course on law, policy, and ethics should definitely be required. In fact, the *Essentials* (AACN, 2006) document recognizes that varying levels of depth in content are needed, depending on the role the DNP will assume following graduation.

The *Consensus Model for APRN Regulation*, published by the National Council of State Boards of Nursing (NCSBN, 2008) and focusing entirely on the four clinical areas of practice (anesthesia, nurse-midwifery, clinical nurse specialists, and nurse practitioners), concurs with the AACN commitment to requiring separate, advanced courses in physiology/pathophysiology, health assessment, and pharmacology. However, additional content related to role and the population to be served "should be integrated throughout the other role and population didactic and clinical courses" (p. 10). The *Consensus Model* (NCSBN, 2008) does not address whether the graduate degree should be at the doctoral level, which may be why its expectation of the level of understanding of the graduate is "comprehensive and at the graduate level" (p. 10), rather than the in-depth level of understanding expected of DNP graduates.

Stanley (2009) underscores the importance of comprehensive education for advanced practice registered nurses (APRNs) as espoused in the *Consensus Model* (NCSBN, 2008). She points out the expectation that NPs would need to be educated and certified to serve adults across the entire age range, so their education would prepare them both as adult and gerontology NPs. The purpose of shifting to the broader scope of practice, according to Stanley (2009), was the increasing needs of the older population. "After extensive national dialogue, the decision to define the population as Adult-Gerontology was made to increase the number of NPs and other APRNs highly prepared to care for the growing older population" (p. 102). So the comprehensive approach to educating APRNs for clinical roles seemed most appropriate. With adequate preparation of faculty to address legal, ethical, and policy matters, these topics could be addressed sufficiently for the breadth of education needed for APRNs. Whether this preparation would be adequate at the doctoral level, however, to prepare the graduate to assume leadership in policy arenas is questionable, and should be studied following implementation of the new regulatory and educational approaches.

RESEARCH APPROACHES FOR UNDERSTANDING THE LAW AND ADVANCED PRACTICE NURSING ROLES

Research addressing ethics questions draws upon traditional social science methods, and is published in journals such as the *Journal of Clinical Ethics*, and in research journals addressing specified foci, such as gerontology or child health care. However, the search for legal principles and decisions requires employment of the legal research method, a method used by legal scholars and lawyers in practice, as well as legislative aides and other policy writers inside and outside government. The legal research method is taught in law schools as a requirement, as is legal writing. Just as nursing practice is based on evidence derived through research, legal practice requires use of evidence derived from legal research, "a process of identifying the rules that govern an activity and finding materials that explain those rules" (Cohen & Olson, 2007, p. 1). Legal research is a qualitative, archival search for legal authority, both primary and secondary. Primary sources are those that are pronouncements from governmental bodies, "court decisions, legislation, and regulations that form the basis of the legal doctrine" (Cohen & Olson, 2007, p. 7). Secondary sources analyze and discuss the primary authority, and assist the researcher to find primary authority. They are used in legal decisions at times to support or explain a particular position taken by a judge.

As a qualitative method, legal research demonstrates both hermeneutic and phenonmenological characteristics (Kjervik, 1995; Kjervik & King, 1990). Legal research requires interpretation of text, as does hermeneutics, to facilitate the understanding of the intended meaning of the words. "Hermeneutic analysis in the legal domain involves consideration of legal trends over time, patterns among legal authorities, paradoxical elements, and objectivity or subjectivity in reasoning and decisions made" (Kjervik, 1995, p. 45). Phenomenology studies the lived experience of an individual. "Legal research seeks to describe the phenomenon of person to person (civil law) or person to state (criminal law) conflict including description and analysis of the writer of the opinion whether it be a judge, a legislature, or an attorney general" (Kjervik & King, 1990, p. 217). In studies using traditional social science methods, a framework for testing assumptions is developed prior to administering surveys or interviews. The framework is referred to as a conceptual framework in quantitative studies, and either conceptual or sensitizing framework in qualitative studies that do not examine detailed statistical tests. As Miles and Huberman (1994) say, "A conceptual framework explains, either graphically or in narrative form, the main things to be studied—the key factors, constructs or variables—and the presumed relationships among them. Frameworks can be rudimentary or elaborate, theory-driven or commonsensical, descriptive or causal" (p. 18). To examine legal phenomena, variables representing these phenomena should be included in the framework so as to test their connections to the other variables in the study. Examples of legal variables are guardianship status, informed consent expressions, dates of statutory enactments, and malpractice judgments by a court.

Legal authorities, such as judges and legislators, use other forms of empirical research in support of their analyses, such as quantitative economic predictions of the value of a loss of a limb or life, statistical analysis of impact of discriminatory practices on the protected class of persons, or descriptive, qualitative predictions of violence from experts. This information is conveyed to legal authorities by expert witnesses in court or persons testifying in legislative hearings. Nurses in practice, nurse researchers, and nursing educators provide testimony in these venues as experts who the law relies upon for their information and decisions. These witnesses provide evidence of facts in health care situations, judgments of the standards of care, and expertise based upon their research findings. Nursing organizations also provide amicus briefs (friend of the court briefs) to inform the judge of their thoughts and opinions about the case. For instance, TAANA offered an amicus brief to the Illinois Supreme Court in the *Sullivan v. Edward Hospital* case (Butler, 2004), in which TAANA argued that only nurses should testify on the standard of care for nurses. The court cited the TAANA brief, stated that it was a persuasive argument, and expressly agreed with it.

Another type of empirical analysis that is useful to legal scholars is legal archeology and feminist legal theory (Threedy, 2008). This type of qualitative research examines one case involving gender issues in depth, using thick, contextual description. It resonates with the ethics orientation, casuistry, in that it examines each case individually and, "can provide insights into systemic weaknesses and vulnerabilities in our system of justice" (Threedy, 2008, p. 172). This approach is also similar to case study research that "investigates a contemporary phenomenon within its real-life context, especially when the boundaries between the phenomenon and context are not clearly evident" (Yin, 1994, p. 13). Theory is generated and tested using an analysis from specific to general propositions. APNs who have information about clinical cases and corresponding legal issues that arise can use this method, as well as others, to conduct research or participate in the research process.

SUMMARY

Educating APNs about legal analysis and requirements involves testing theories and using this evidence to prepare themselves to understand both legal and ethical underpinnings of the law and to become policy advocates for patients, families, and communities. DNPs are most likely to assume the roles of policy analyst and advocate for change and, thus, need in-depth preparation of the substance of law as specified in the TAANA model curriculum (Brooke et al., 2003), legal research method, and the use of other types of research that are commonly used in legal forums.

Understanding the connection between law and nursing theory provides the conceptual landscape in which testing legal, ethical, and nursing phenomena together can take place. Recognizing the intersection between law, ethics, and nursing will provide a powerful tool for change that will be evidence-based and contain interdisciplinary strength. APNs are practice leaders in nursing, and with legal and ethical sophistication, will be well positioned to meet and argue persuasively in support of their commitments to the public and to the nursing discipline.

KEY POINTS

1. Law is a gatekeeper in the process of changing the status of APNs and their work environments.

2. Connecting legal realities to the study of APN practice will give APNs the tools to advocate most effectively for their patients and the profession.
3. Policy leadership is expected of Doctors of Nursing Practice.
4. Legal research methods should be employed to obtain the clearest possible understanding of the law.
5. Law and nursing theory together provide the conceptual basis for testing the efficacy of APN policy choices related to practice outcomes.

REFERENCES

American Academy of Nurse Practitioners. (2007). *Position statement on nurse practitioner curriculum*. Retrieved April 18, 2010, from http://www.aanp.org/NR/rdonlyres/59523729-0179-466A-A7FB-BDEE68160E8E/0/NPCurriculum.pdf

American Association of Colleges of Nursing. (2006, October). *The essentials of doctoral education for advanced nursing practice*. Retrieved from http://www.aacn.nche.edu/DNP/pdf/Essentials.pdf

American Association of Colleges of Nursing. (2009, April). *Fact sheet: The doctor of nursing practice (DNP)*. Retrieved August 11, 2009 from http://www.aacn.nche.edu/Media/pdf/FS_dnp.pdf

Boyer, E. (1990). *Scholarship reconsidered: Priorities of the professoriate*. Princeton, NJ: Carnegie Foundation for the Advancement of Teaching.

Brooke, P., Badzek, L., Auton, L., Killion, S., Kjervik, D., & Weaver, J. (2003). *Model curriculum of legal content in nursing education* (2nd ed.). Pensacola, FL: The American Association of Nurse Attorneys.

Butler, K. (2004). Interest of amici curiae brief: Submitted in support of respondent, *Sullivan v. Edward Hospital*, Illinois Supreme Court. *Journal of Nursing Law, 9*(4), 6–14.

Cohen, M. L., & Olson, K. C. (2007). *Legal research in a nutshell*. (9th ed.). St. Paul, MN: Thomson/West.

Kjervik, D. (1995). The hermeneutics of nursing law research. *Journal of Nursing Law, 2*(3), 39–47.

Kjervik, D., & King, F. E. (1990), The legal research method: An approach to enhance nursing science. *Journal of Professional Nursing, 6*(4), 213–220.

Kleffel, D. (2006), The evolution of the environmental paradigm of nursing. In L. C. Andrist, P. K. Nicolas, & K. A. Wolf (Eds.), *A history of nursing ideas*. Boston: Jones and Bartlett.

Majchrzak, A. (1984). *Methods for policy research*. Newbury Park, CA: Sage.

Miles, M. B., & Huberman, A. M. (1994). *Qualitative data analysis* (2nd ed.). Thousand Oaks, CA: Sage.

National Council of State Boards of Nursing. (2008, July) *Consensus model for APRN regulation: Licensure, accreditation, certification and education*. Retrieved April 18, 2010, from https://www.ncsbn.org/7_23_08_Consensue_APRN_Final.pdf

National Organization of Nurse Practitioner Faculties. (n.d.) *Sample curriculum templates for practice doctorate NP education*. Retrieved April 18, 2010, from http://www.nonpf.org/NONPF2005/Buttons/DNP-NPCurricTemplates0907.pdf

Numminen, O., Arend, A., & Leino-Kilpi, H. (2009). Nurse educators' and nursing students' perspectives on teaching codes of ethics. *Nursing Ethics, 16*(1), 69–82.

Pappas, I. E., Clutter, L. B., & Maggi, E. (2007). Current legal changes: Innovative legal seminar for nursing student. *Journal of Nursing Law, 11*(4), 197–209.

Pierce, S. T. (2005). Integrating evidence-based practice into nursing curricula. In M. H. Oermann & K. T. Heinrich (Eds.), *Annual review of nursing education: Strategies for teaching, assessment, and program planning.* New York: Springer Publishing Company.

Stanley, J. (2009). Reaching consensus on a regulatory model: What does this mean for APRNs? *Journal for Nurse Practitioners, 5*(2), 99–104.

Threedy, D. L. (2008). Legal archeology and feminist legal theory: A case study of gender and domestic violence. *Women's Rights Law Reporter, 29*(4), 171–192.

Wexler, D. B., & Winick, B. J. (1996). *Law in a therapeutic key.* Durham, NC: Carolina Academic Press.

White, J. (2006). Patterns of knowing: Review, critique, and update. In L. C. Andrist, P. K. Nicolas, & K. A. Wolf (Eds.), *A history of nursing ideas.* Boston: Jones and Bartlett.

Yeo, M. (1997). Integration of nursing theory and nursing ethics. In L. H. Nicoll (Ed.), *Perspectives on nursing theory* (3rd ed.). Philadelphia: Lippincott.

Yin, R. K. (1994). *Case study research: Design and methods* (2nd ed.). Thousand Oaks, CA: Sage.

TABLE OF CASES

Sullivan v. Edward Hospital, 209 Ill.2d. 100, 806 N.E.2d. 645, 282 Ill.Dec. 348 (2004).

8 International Law and Nurses

EDITH ANN BROUS AND GINA RAINERI BERNAIN

The most promising strategy for achieving international balance in health workforce resources is for each country to have an adequate and sustainable source of health professionals.

—Linda Aiken

INTRODUCTION

Failure to address correctable problems lies at the core of the global nursing shortage. Intolerable working conditions accelerate the pace of migration. Nurses in poorer countries are pushed to emigrate in search of better and safer living conditions for themselves and their families (Khaliq, Broyles, & Mwachofi, 2009)). Attempts to reduce or ban emigration from these countries will be unsuccessful, because they neglect the underlying cause of the exodus. Providing adequate employment opportunities, sustainable salaries, and safe practice environments would be a more effective approach.

The wealthier countries have shortages, in large part, because nurses who are qualified to practice choose not to do so (Salmon & Guisinger, 2007). Industrialized, developed countries address staffing deficiencies by seeking nurses from overseas, rather than addressing the underlying causes of their own shortages, as is evidenced by findings such as: more than 500,000 nurses in the United States are not actively employed (Padilla, 2006), Ireland has 15,000 nurses unwilling to work in the current system (Oulton, 2007), and South Africa has more than 35,000 unemployed nurses (Solidarity Research Institute, 2009).

Multiple factors have contributed to the shortage in wealthier countries. Demand has increased, whereas supply has been reduced. On the demand side, an aging patient population has created a greater need for nursing care. Shorter inpatient stays have increased the acuity level of hospitalized, outpatient, and home care patients. Technical advances in health care have created greater demand for increasingly higher levels of sophisticated nursing care.

On the supply side, fewer nurses are available to employers. Women, who compromise the vast majority of the nursing workforce, are increasingly taking advantage of the opportunity to participate in career choices previously available only to men. A nursing faculty shortage, coupled with difficulty in providing sufficient clinical practice sites, has reduced the number of qualified applicants who can be accepted into nursing programs. The nursing workforce is aging as the baby boomer generation nears retirement. Stressful working conditions create dissatisfaction, reduce morale, accelerate turnover, and contribute to attrition. Increased workloads and unsafe staffing ratios drive an exodus of providers from the workforce. Workplace dissatisfaction reduces the retention of experienced nurses. As such, novice nurses are not provided adequate orientation and support. This contributes to the dissatisfaction and failure to retain these new nurses, as well.

Relentless portrayals of nurses as uneducated physician extenders, sexualized naughty nurses, or compassionate (but not necessarily educated, skilled, or intelligent) "angels of mercy" demoralize those in clinical practice. Pervasive media imagery of nurses in such a disrespectful and inaccurate light deters others from considering nursing as a career. Anachronistic depictions of nurses serve as a disincentive to entering or remaining in the nursing workforce (Buresh & Gordon, 2006).

Economic globalization and universal nursing shortages have combined to make the international migration of nurses a multi-billion dollar industry (Padilla, 2006). As Dr. Buchan notes, "[I]nternational recruitment is big business. There is a lot of money at stake for this particular issue" (Buchan, 2006, p. 23s). Some countries intentionally produce nurses for the express purpose of exportation in the same manner as fungible goods. A 2002 study, for example, demonstrated that approximately 85% of employed Philippine nurses were working abroad (Lorenzo, Galvez-Tan, Icamina, & Javier, 2007). As nurses become business commodities, the potential for exploitation is great.

This chapter will describe some of the legal and ethical issues related to international law and nursing, with special focus on the international migration of nurses. It will begin with a brief survey of the differences between major legal systems to provide context for the discussion.

SOURCES OF LAW

Common law, civil law, socialist law, and Islamic law are examples of the types of systems that exist throughout the world. They present ideological and philosophical diversity in their approach to conflict resolution. Although there are fundamental differences among them, the distinctions have become less pronounced and convergence more common. Some countries use a combination of one or the other of these schemes, and other countries use one of these systems in combination with religious, tribal, military (martial), socialist, or other traditional structures (Butty, 2005).

Civil Law

Civil law is sometimes referred to as "European," "Romano-Germanic," or "Continental" law, and is the system used in France, Germany, Austria, Greece, Brazil, Portugal, Turkey, Japan, South Korea, Taiwan, Mexico, Haiti, Bolivia, Chile, Ecuador, Uruguay, Argentina, Columbia, Peru, Denmark, Finland, Iceland, Norway, Sweden, and Switzerland, among other countries.

This legal system dates back to Roman law and is the oldest form of jurisprudence. It is based on a codified system of statutes in which the codes, rather than judicial opinions, determine the outcome of a case. The ancient Code of Hammurabi is thought to be the first such codification of law. A strict separation of powers restricts the source of law to the legislature or executive branch. Judges may only apply the law as promulgated through the legislature, or the regulations as promulgated by the executive branch. Court decisions do not have the authority to bind future courts through the concept of precedence. The Napoleonic Code is an example of civil law.

Civil law jurisdictions analyze cases by focusing on the written law and applying its principles. Previous cases do not serve as a source of authority for decisions. The law is more rigid, as it can only be changed by the legislature. In criminal cases, the civil law system may be more inquisitorial than adversarial. There may or may not be a presumption of innocence or the right to a jury trial.

Common Law

United States jurisprudence (with the exception of Louisiana) is based on the British Commonwealth system, also called the "Anglo-Saxon" system or the "English common law" system. Among other countries, this system is used in England, Wales, Ghana, Cameroon, Ireland, Australia, New Zealand, Pakistan, India, Hong Kong, Belgium, Luxemburg, Singapore, Italy, Spain, and most of Canada.

The common law system may be referred to as "judge-made law," and is based on precedent. Rules are created from specific cases, referred to as case law. The body of case law dates back to the Norman conquest of England in 1066. In the traditional English system, judges (called lords) heard arguments by prosecutors (called solicitors) and defense counsel (called barristers) to determine the truth in a particular dispute. It was, and remains, an adversarial system.

There were originally two distinct types of courts. One was a court of law, in which the judges applied written statutes to the cases. The other type was a court of equity, in which no statutes covered the situation. In the absence of written statutes, judges in these cases established the law by writing opinions that became binding on future court decisions involving similar issues. The courts of law and courts of equity have totally merged in some states. Some states have separate law and equity divisions in the same courts. Yet other states retain separate courts for law and equity.

Common law jurisdictions analyze cases by focusing on the specific facts of the matter and applying the rules as determined in previous cases. It is less rigid than the law in civil jurisdictions, as it is capable of change through judicial decisions. In criminal cases, the defendant is presumed innocent until proven guilty and is guaranteed the right to a trial by jury.

Mixed Jurisdictions

Louisiana jurisprudence is based on a mixture of both common law and civil law, as is Quebec, Scotland, the Philippines, Mauritius, Sri Lanka, Puerto Rico, St. Lucia, the Seychelles, Zimbabwe, Nicaragua, Namibia, Israel, Lesotho, Swaziland, and South Africa. These "mixed jurisdictions," as they are referred to, are hybrid systems that demonstrate features of both common law and civil law. Similarly, international law is an evolving system of jurisprudence with the dual characteristics of both the common law and civil law structures.

INTERNATIONAL ISSUES

Recruitment

Nurses who are enlisted to leave their home countries for work abroad may have no experience and/or education in the ethics and legalities of recruitment. They may be asked to pay exorbitant fees in excess of what the sponsor facilities have already paid to the recruiting agency, and in violation of the laws of many countries. They may be misled or overtly lied to about the employing facilities, hours, shifts, pay scale, working conditions, living arrangements, or other contract terms. Critical documents, such as passports, visas, identification papers, or custom and immigration records may be held hostage to the recruiting agency's demands. Arrival in the host country may present many unpleasant surprises. Nurses, primarily women, may not know their rights or where to obtain assistance with untenable situations. A case frequently referred to as "The Sentosa 27" serves as an example of this type of exploitation.

Sentosa, a Philippine-based recruitment agency, recruited 1 physical therapist and 26 nurses to work in the United States. The nurses signed direct-hire individual employment contracts for specific nursing homes, with the understanding that they would be working in those sponsoring facilities. The contracts obligated them to work for 3 years and provided for liquidated damages in the amount of $25,000 should they fail to honor that commitment. They were told that temporary permits had been obtained, and they would be working as registered nurses immediately upon arrival while permanent New York licenses were pending. They were promised reimbursement for licensure expenses and plane fare, in addition to 2 months of free housing.

Upon arrival, they found themselves to be employees of Sentosa Services (doing business as Prompt Nursing Employment Agency), not of the nursing homes, and were assigned to facilities other than those with which they had signed agreements. Temporary permits had not been obtained, making it impossible to work as nurses. To support themselves, some of the nurses worked in clerical positions at substantially lower pay than they had been promised. They were not paid for the hours they actually worked, nor were they paid shift differentials, overtime, holiday pay, or agreed-to hourly rates. Reimbursement and free housing were also not forthcoming for all of the nurses. Some nurses' green cards were initially held by Sentosa. Additionally, they were housed in substandard conditions.

The nurses complained about these contract violations, and identified patient safety issues presented by insufficient orientation and inadequate staffing. When the complaints were not addressed, they sought the assistance of the New York State Nurses Association, the Philippine Labor Attache's Office, and the Consulate General. They were referred to Felix Vinluan, an attorney with expertise in immigration and labor law. Mr. Vinluan filed a complaint on their behalf with the Office of Special Counsel for Immigration Related Unfair Employment Practices in Washington, DC. He also filed an administrative complaint with the Philippine Overseas Employment Administration (POEA) for violations of Philippine recruitment regulations. The POEA administrator signed a preventive suspension order against Sentosa, which was lifted after the intervention of Senator Charles Schumer.

The nurses feared retaliation during any period between the date of giving notice and the effective date of their resignations. As such, they collectively resigned at the end of their shifts or in advance of their next shifts, providing between 8 and 72 hours notice. At the time of their resignations, the nurses were aware that Sentosa had replacement nurses available.

Their fears of retaliation were well founded, as Sentosa responded to the resignations by filing breach-of-contract suits and reporting them to the nursing board with allegations of patient abandonment. Additionally, Sentosa requested a private meeting with Suffolk County District Attorney Thomas Spota, requesting that he investigate the nurses. The nursing board ultimately closed the investigation, finding that there had been no abandonment or moral character issues, and advising Mr. Vinluan that there would be no prohibition on issuance of permits or licenses on that basis. Approximately 1 year after the resignations, Mr. Spota, a recipient of political campaign contributions from Sentosa's lawyers, filed a criminal complaint against 10 of the nurses and Mr. Vinluan. They were indicted on 13 counts of conspiracy and endangering the welfare of children and disabled persons.

The nurses and Mr. Vinluan attempted to have the criminal indictments dismissed, arguing that the prosecutions violated their constitutional rights. They commenced a proceeding to prohibit Mr. Spota from prosecuting them, claiming that the prosecution infringed on their First, Thirteenth, and Fourteenth Amendment rights. The First Amendment states, in part, "Congress shall make no law...abridging the freedom of speech...." The Thirteenth Amendment states, in part, "Neither slavery nor involuntary servitude, except as a punishment for crime whereof the party shall have been duly convicted, shall exist within the United States, or any place subject to their jurisdiction." The Fourteenth Amendment states, in part, "No State shall make or enforce any law which shall abridge the privileges or immunities of citizens of the United States; nor shall any State deprive any person of life, liberty, or property, without due process of law; nor deny to any person within its jurisdiction the equal protection of the laws" (United States Constitution).

The nurses contended that the prosecution was legal coercion that compelled them to work against their will. Criminal sanctions for resigning effectively subjected them to involuntary servitude (in violation of the Thirteenth Amendment). The Court agreed and granted the petition to prohibit the prosecution:

> [T]he indictment handed down against the petitioners explicitly makes the nurses' conduct in resigning their positions a component of each of the crimes charged. Thus, the indictment places the nurses in the position of being required to remain in Sentosa's service after submitting their resignations, even if only for a relatively brief period of notice, or being subject to criminal sanction. Accordingly, the prosecution has the practical effect of exposing the nurses to criminal penalty for exercising their right to leave their employment at will. The imposition of such a limitation upon the nurses' ability to freely exercise their right to resign from the service of an employer who allegedly failed to fulfill the promises and commitments made to them is the antithesis of the free and voluntary system of labor envisioned by the framers of the Thirteenth Amendment.-...Furthermore, the prosecution impermissibly violates Vinluan's constitutionally protected rights of expression and association in violation of the First and Fourteenth Amendments. It cannot be doubted that an attorney has a constitutional right to provide legal advice to his clients within the bounds of the law. (*Vinluan v. Doyle*, 2009, pp. 248, 250)

Subsequent to the court decision in this matter, the Philippine National Labor Relations Commission (NLRC) found that the Sentosa-affiliated facilities had substantially breached the nurses' employment contracts, and issued a decision ordering Sentosa Recruitment Agency and the various nursing home facilities that contracted with the nurses to pay the nurses more than $186,000 in actual damages for nonpayment or underpayment of salaries and benefits.

The Sentosa 27 case illustrates the perils to which migrating nurses may be subject. Although not transported for the purposes of sexual exploitation, the ethical and legal violations in this case may rise to the level of human trafficking. The recruitment, transportation, and subsequent threat of criminal prosecution of these nurses may constitute exploitation for manual labor. The United Nations Convention against Transnational Organized Crime defines human trafficking as:

> The action of recruitment, transportation, transfer, harbouring or receipt of persons, by means of the threat or use of force or other forms of coercion, abduction, fraud, deception, abuse of power or vulnerability or payments or benefits to achieve the consent of a person for the purposes of exploitation. Forms of exploitation include but are not limited to the exploitation of the prostitution of others, sexual exploitation, forced labour or services, slavery or similar practices, servitude and the removal of organs. (United Nations Office on Drugs and Crime, 2007, p. 2)

The depletion of health care providers from resource-poor countries for the advantage of resource-rich countries raises ethical concerns. This "brain drain," as it has been called, has global public health implications.

Danger

International migration can also pose safety issues for nurses. In addition to cultural and language differences, the laws and legal systems of the destination countries may be significantly unlike those of the nurse's home country. This was dramatically illustrated in 1999 in Libya.

In the late 1990s, the AIDS crisis in Libya drew public scrutiny after a media exposé revealed an epidemic infection rate at El-Fatih Children's Hospital in Benghazi. The AIDS outbreak included over 400 children. In February of 1999, 23 foreign health care professionals (HCPs) working in Libya were detained. In March of 1999, six of those workers were arrested, including five Bulgarian nurses and one Palestinian physician. The "Benghazi Six," as they came to be called, were accused by Muammar al-Gaddafi of working with the United States Central Intelligence Agency (CIA) and with the Israeli national intelligence agency (Mossad) to intentionally infect Libyan children.

In response to Libya's request for assistance, the World Health Organization (WHO) sent a team of doctors to Tripoli. They determined that the HIV virus had been accidently transmitted from the re-use of syringes and medical equipment, as well as inadequate sterilization. DNA studies indicated that the genetic antecedent of the strains of HIV with which the children were infected had been in existence a full year before the arrival of the health care workers (Butler, 2006). The source of the infection was thought to be a patient with multiple admissions between 1994 and 1997.

The HCPs were charged with murder, threatening the security of the state, and causing an epidemic. They were also charged with violating Islamic law by drinking alcohol, "illegally transacting in foreign currency," and engaging in nonmarital sexual relations. They were also accused of conspiring with the CIA and Mossad to conduct experiments on the children. Although the International Council of Nurses (ICN) had called for a just, fair, and expeditious trial, confessions were obtained through torture and threats against the health care workers' families (ICN, 2006; Rosenthal, 2005; Truthout, 2006). Despite the WHO expert reports, the health care workers were tried, convicted of intentionally infecting 429 children, and sentenced to death by firing squad. The Libyan Supreme Court retried them, upholding the conviction and the death penalty.

The ICN issued press releases condemning the death sentences, calling for action on the trial (International Council of Nurses, 2004), and calling for justice (International Council of Nurses, 2007), as did Amnesty International (2006), the Council of Europe Parliamentary Assembly (2005, 2007), and other nongovernmental organizations. The ICN also issued joint press releases with the World Medical Association (WMA) pleading to drop the death sentences (International Council of Nurses, 2006). Upon appeal to the High Judicial Council (Libya's highest court), the sentence was converted from death to life imprisonment on July 17, 2007. The ICN (2005) and WMA issued another joint press release welcoming the court's decision to reverse the death sentence.

In attempting to negotiate their freedom, the European Union (EU) offered to provide medical equipment, HIV treatment, and humanitarian aid. The EU sent medical teams to Libya to assist in the country's AIDS epidemic, conducted training programs for Libyan physicians, and transported many of the children to Europe for treatment. Bulgaria wrote off almost $57 million of Libya's debt (Republic of Bulgaria Council of Ministers, 2007).

Libyan officials responded by demanding $10 million for each of the 420 children they claimed had been infected. (This is the same amount Libya had agreed to pay to the 270 families of the people killed in Pan Am Flight 103 bombing over Lockerbie, Scotland.) Libya also demanded that Bulgaria make payments to the children's families. Under Islamic law, the families would then be permitted to forgive the health care workers and ask Libya to dismiss the charges. Bulgaria rejected such demands as "blood money" payments, not permitted or accepted under Bulgarian law. An agreement was reached in which $461 million was to be given to the Benghazi International Fund (Gaddaffi, 2006; *Tripoli Post*, 2007).

A prisoner exchange agreement was used in the negotiations, such that Libya would not pardon or release the prisoners, but would permit them to serve their life sentences in Bulgaria. On July 24, 2007, after 8 years in prison, the health care workers were extradited to Bulgaria to serve their sentences. Upon arrival, Bulgarian President Georgi Parvanov pardoned them (Radio Free Europe, 2007).

The ICN and WMA again issued a joint press release welcoming this news (ICN, 2007). Predeparture classes for migrating nurses may assist them in preparing for overseas work and reduce the danger in doing so. Such classes should address the laws and customs of the destination countries by which they have been recruited.

The Chilean Perspective

Centuries before the first Spanish physician set foot on Chilean soil, the indigenous Mapuche people conducted extravagant healing ceremonies, called Machitún. Prior to the Spanish conquest, the aboriginal women of Chile were dedicated to the care and healing of the sick. They had no professional training. Inés de Saurez came from Peru with the conquistadores and assisted in the founding of Santiago de Chile. The expedition had no physician, and she herself set fractures and healed wounds. During the early years of the conquest, medicine developed as a mixture of indigenous Hispanic medicine, primitive methods, and religious ritual in the absence of European physicians or hospitals.

In the years following the arrival of the Spanish, European doctors arrived in Chile, followed by Dominican and Jesuit missionaries. Universities and hospitals were founded and influenced by military surgery and medical reform. Women worked as healers, phlebotomists, bleeders, and midwives. Healers gave way to nurses who still had no formal education until 1902, when the first course of nursing study was taught at the de Hospital de Niños Roberto del Río. The first hospital school of nursing was created in 1906, and the first baccalaureate program was established in 1937 at the Universidad de Chile.

The National Health Service (Sistema Nacional de Servicios de Salud—SNSS) is the successor of the original 1952 public health service, and remains the largest health care provider in the country. This was followed by the creation in 1953 of the first nursing board. By 2001, the president of the Chilean nurses association was serving as a member of the International Council of Nursing, representing South America.

Currently, the Chilean health care system is a mixed system of the National Health Service public system (SNSS), providing approximately 70% of the nation's health care, and the private sector, providing the remaining 30%. Despite being one of the best-performing health systems in the region, the SNSS faces a serious staffing crisis caused by a deficit of nurses willing to work in the public sector. Although the SNSS is attempting to improve health care through Care Management and a family health model, it is not competitive with the private sector. There is, therefore, an internal migration within the country of nurses from the public to the private sector and from the rural to the urban centers.

The resultant staffing shortages have forced the SNSS to use non-nurses in the provision of nursing care. As the Pan American Health Organization (PAHO) notes, "The practices or fields that have traditionally been the responsibility of nursing, especially those related to health promotion and disease prevention, have been taken over by professionals from other disciplines, in most cases without the necessary academic preparation" (Pan American Health Organization, 2004, p. 16). Despite the strong midwifery care and services model that exists in Chile, poor working conditions and the lack of prestige or professional status for nurses and midwives perpetuate the shortage (Pan American Health Organization, 2004, p. 15).

Although nursing provides 90% of pediatric and well-baby care, Chile's public health sector patients are satisfied with the care they provide; positive outcomes and shorter hospital stays are associated with the provision of nursing case management, and the services nursing provides are less expensive with the same technical quality of general practitioners; there is little nursing presence in the government's health care decision-making process (Pan American Health Organization, 2004, pp. 1–2). Similarly, although 99.8% of deliveries in Chile occur in public or private health care facilities assisted by midwives and/or midwife nurses, there are very few nursing midwife publications in national journals, and none appear in indexed journals (Fernandez, 2006, pp. 2–4).

As primary health care providers, Chilean nurses and midwives reduce morbidity and mortality and strengthen the health of the country's population. Their ability to remain effective requires that they also be involved in high-level decision making, policy development, and public health strategic planning. In recognition of this as a global issue, the World Health Assembly in May 2002 adopted resolution 54.12, Strengthening Nursing and Midwifery:

Recognising the importance of using appropriate resources, including human resources, in the provision of health services; Recognising the importance of nursing services and midwifery services being the core of any health system and in national health; Aware that nurses and midwives play a crucial role in reducing excess mortality, morbidity and disability and in promoting healthy lifestyles. (World Health Assembly, 2001)

Member states were asked to involve nurses and midwives in the framing, planning, and implementation of health policy, review and develop models of education, legislation, regulation, and practice for nurses and midwives, develop human resource plans that support training, recruitment, and retention, ensure healthy workplaces for nurses and midwives, continuously assess nursing and midwifery plans, and enhance the development of nursing and midwifery services based on evidence.

Health care reform efforts in Chile have tackled multiple issues. The government has invested in medical equipment and nursing education. A lack of participation by patients in their own health care has been addressed by mandating that they play a part in their own health and educating them as health care consumers. Cost-containment and quality issues have been addressed, along with efforts to decentralize care and reduce the disparities. Funding for primary health services to benefit the poor and salary increases in the public sector have attempted to improve public health. What remains is to recognize nursing and midwifery as the critical link in the delivery of services. Additionally, working conditions and critical workforce shortages must be addressed to maintain adequate staffing and stem the exodus of providers. Nurses and midwives in Chile must be involved at the national and local levels in strategic planning and decision making.

Solutions

In recognition of the critical role nurses play in public health, the WHO (WHO), the PAHO, and the ICN have impressed upon governments the need to strengthen the health systems in which nurses work. Particularly in the Americas, these organizations have recommended that a strategic plan of action be adopted to focus on nursing and midwifery.

The World Trade Organization's General Agreement on Trade Services (GATS) requires that government measures not be overly burdensome, such that they restrain trade in service. Although nursing regulators in destination countries maintain their sovereignty, they must be mindful of trade agreements (Hellquist & Nissen, n.d.).

The ICN issued a position statement on ethical nurse recruitment in 2001, in which it recognized that in depleting source countries of their nurses, international migration may compromise health care quality in those countries. It called for mechanisms to assist migrating nurses who wish to return to their home countries. The ICN also called for destination countries to address the issues that contribute to their own shortages. In denouncing unethical recruitment practices, the ICN called for regulation in the recruitment process (ICN, 2001). Such regulation and oversight may reduce abuses such as those described in the Sentosa and Benghazi matters. The ICN also joined forces with the Commission on Graduates of Foreign Nursing Schools (CGFNS) in 2005 to form the International Centre on Nurse Migration. The Center was established to address issues in the migrant nursing workforce.

SUMMARY

Universally, nurses and advanced practice nurses are the backbone of health care. A critical shortage of nursing providers compromises public health. Disparities are intensified when resource-rich countries recruit nurses from resource-poor countries. Migration occurs from nation to nation, and within a country from the public to the private sector. Addressing workplace issues, working conditions, salaries, prestige, and ethical recruitment practices must be the focus of all countries and of the international community. In the eloquent words of Commonwealth Steering Committee for Nursing and Midwifery:

> As was agreed in adopting resolution WHA 54.12, we believe that all nations should act to strengthen nursing and midwifery services. As we acknowledge our interdependence on this planet, all partners must work together in their stewardship role to improve the health of populations globally. (Wold, McQuide, Golden, Maslin, & Salmon, 2003, p. 9)

KEY POINTS

1. Working conditions must be improved to maintain adequate nursing workforces in all practice settings and countries.
2. Until and unless all recruiting agencies engage in ethical recruiting practices, nurses must be extremely cautious in entering agreements, and carefully research the agencies.

3. Nurses who migrate must consider the legal system of the host county and how it differs from their own.
4. Organizations such as the International Council of Nurses may provide resources and support.
5. Advanced-practice nurses, particularly midwives, play a critical role in global public health and must be visible and active players locally, nationally, and internationally in formulation of health policy.

REFERENCES

Aiken, L., Buchan, J., Sochalski, J., Nichols, B., & Powell, M. (2004). Trends in international nurse migration. *Health Affairs, 23*, 3, 69–77. Retrieved April 15, 2010, from http://content.healthaffairs.org/cgi/reprint/23/3/69

Amnesty International. (2006, July 19). *Press release: Libya: Death sentences for foreign medics must be withdrawn.* Retrieved September 3, 2009, from http://www.amnestyusa.org/document.php?id=ENGMDE190072006&lang=e

Buresh, B., & Gordon, S. (2006). *From silence to voice: What nurses know and must communicate to the public* (2nd ed.). Ithaca, NY: ILR Press.

Buchan, J. (2006). The impact of global nursing migration on health services delivery. *Policy, Politics, & Nursing Practice, 7*(3, Suppl.), 16s–25s.

Butler, D. (2006, September 21). Lawyers call for science to clear AIDS nurses in Libya, international pressure needed to save health workers from death penalty. *Nature, 442*, 254. Retrieved September 3, 2009, from http://www.nature.com/nature/journal/v443/n7109/full/443254b.html

Butty, V., based on a text by Fleiner, T. (2005). *Common law and continental law: Two legal systems.* Retrieved September 2, 2009, from http://www.federalism.ch/files/documents/legalsystems_tipsheet_20 9.02_final.pdf

Council of Europe Parliamentary Assembly. (2005). *Recommendation 1726, serious human rights violations in Libya—Inhuman treatment of Bulgarian medical staff.* Retrieved September 3, 2009, from http://assembly.coe.int/Main.asp?link=/Documents/AdoptedText/ta05 /EREC1726.htm

European Union. (2007). *European Parliament resolution on the imprisonment and trial of five Bulgarian nurses and a Palestinian doctor on charges related to the 1999 HIV/ AIDS case at the Benghazi Children's Hospital.* Retrieved September 3, 2009, from http://www.europarl.europa.eu/sides/getDoc.do?type=MOTION&reference=B6-2007 -0028&language=EN

Fernandez, P. (2006). *Newborn care in Chile.* Retrieved December 18, 2009, from http:// www.coinnurses.org/newsletters/doc/2006/june06.pdf

Gaddaffi International Charity and Development Foundation. (2006). *Press release about the meeting of Benghazi International Fund Board of Directors and representatives of the Families' Association for Benghazi Children Infected With AIDS.* Retrieved September 3, 2009, from http://gdf.org.ly/index.php?lang=ar&CAT_NO=4&DATA_NO =85&MAIN_CAT_ NO=4&Page=105&lang=en

Hellquist, K., & Nissen, T. (n.d.). *Global trade agreements: What do nurse regulators need to know and how this impacts the overseas applicant?* Retrieved December 18, 2009, from https://www.ncsbn.org/ICN_Poster(3).pdf

International Council of Nurses. (1997, July 24). *Joint press release with the World Medical Association: ICN and WMA welcome the release of Bulgarian nurses and*

Palestinian physician. Retrieved September 3, 2009, from http://www.icn.ch/PR19 _07.htm

International Council of Nurses. (2001). *Position statement: Ethical nurse recruitment.* Retrieved December 18, 2009, from http://www.icn.ch/psrecruit01.htm

International Council of Nurses. (2004, May 8). *Press release: International Council of Nurses condemns Libyan death sentence of Bulgarian nurses, Palestinian physician.* Retrieved September 3, 2009, from http://www.icn.ch/PR04_04.htm

International Council of Nurses. (2005, December 26). *Press release: Nurses and physicians welcome Libyan court's decision to reverse death sentences.* Retrieved September 3, 2009, from http://www.icn.ch/PR24_05.htm

International Council of Nurses. (2006, September 12). *Press release: ICN calls for action on the trial of Bulgarian nurses and Palestinian physician in Libya.* Retrieved September 3, 2009, from http://www.icn.ch/PR14_06.htm

International Council of Nurses. (2006, December 14). *Joint press release with the World Medical Association: WMA and ICN plead to drop death sentences against doctors and nurses after new scientific evidence.* Retrieved September 3, 2009, from http:// www.icn.ch/PR24_06.htm#statement

International Council of Nurses. (2007, May 29). *Joint press release with the World Medical Association: Global nursing caucus calls for justice for Bulgarian nurses, Palestinian doctor and Libyan children.* Retrieved September 3, 2009, from http:// www.icn.ch/PR17_07.htm

Khaliq, A., Broyles, R., & Mwachofi, A. (2009). Global nurse migration: Its impact on developing countries and prospects for the future. *World Health and Population, 10*(3).

Lorenzo, F., Galvez-Tan, J., Icamina, K., & Javier, L. (2007). Nurse migration from a source country perspective: Philippine country case study. *Health Services Research, 42*(3, Pt 2), 1406–1418. Retrieved April 16, 2010, rom http://www.pubmedcentral. nih.gov/articlerender.fcgi?artid=1955369

Oulton, J. (2007). Nursing in the international community: A broader view of nursing issues. *Policy and politics in nursing and health care* (5th ed., pp. 966–981). St. Louis, MO: Saunders Elsevier.

Padilla, P. (2006, April/May). Nurse migration and the nursing shortage. *NSNA Imprint.* Retrieved September 2, 2009, from http://www.nsna.org/pdf/IMPRINT_APRIL06_ BTN.pdf

Pan American Health Organization. (2004). *Nursing and midwifery services contributing to equity, access, coverage, quality, and sustainability in the health services.* Retrieved December 17, 2009, from http://www.paho.org/English/AD/THS/OS/nur-svcs-eng.pdf

Radio Free Europe. (2007, July 24). *Bulgarian medics pardoned after arrival from Libya.* Retrieved September 3, 2009, from http://www.rferl.org/content/article/1077780. html

Republic of Bulgaria Council of Ministers. (2007). *Bulgarian government's humanitarian gesture toward Benghazi International Fund exceeds 55 million US dollars.* Retrieved September 3, 2009, from http://old.government.bg/cgi-bin/e-cms/vis/vis.pl?s=001& p=0137&n= 451&g=

Rosenthal, E. (2005, October 14). Time ebbing for 6 foreigners in Libya AIDS case. *New York Times.* Retrieved September 3, 2009, from http://www.nytimes.com/2005/ 10/14/health/14iht-nurses.html

Salmon, M., & Guisinger, V. (2007). Global migration of nurses: Managing a scarce resource. *Policy and politics in nursing and health care* (5th ed., pp. 982–991). St. Louis, MO: Saunders Elsevier.

Solidarity Research Institute. (2009). *Nurse shortage in South Africa: Nurse/patient ratios report*. Retrieved September 2, 2009, from http://us-cdn.creamermedia.co.za/assets/articles/attachments/2137 3_solidarity.pdf

Tripoli Post. (2007, July 25). EU Commission confirms $461 million fund for Libyan HIV infected children. Retrieved September 3, 2009, from http://www.tripolipost.com/articledetail.asp?c=1&i=1002

Truthout.org. (2006, May 17). Testimony: Bulgarian nurses were tortured in Libya. *Le Nouvel Observateur*. Retrieved September 3, 2009, from http://www.truthout.org/article/testimony-bulgarian-nurses-were-t ortured-libya

United Nations Office on Drugs and Crime. (2007). *Trafficking in persons*. Retrieved September 2, 2009, from http://www.unodc.org/documents/human-trafficking/HT_GPATleaflet07_en.pdf

United States Constitution, First Amendment. Retrieved April 19, 2010, from http://www.usconstitution.net/const.html

United States Constitution, Thirteenth Amendment. Retrieved April 19, 2010, from http://www.usconstitution.net/const.html

United States Constitution, Fourteenth Amendment. Retrieved April 19, 2010, from http://www.usconstitution.net/const.html

Wold, J., McQuide, P., Golden, C., Maslin, A, & Salmon, M. (2003). Caring that counts: The evidence base for the effectiveness of nursing and midwifery interventions. *Commonwealth Steering Committee for Nursing and Midwifery*. Retrieved December 18, 2009, from http://www.amddprogram.org/conference/assets/Resources/Day%201/Task%20Shifting/Lupo%20Wold%20et%20al_Caring%20That%20Counts-Evidence%20for%20Interventions_2003.pdf

World Health Assembly. (2001). *Strengthening nursing and midwifery, Resolution no. 54.12* Retrieved April 15, 2010, from http://www.searo.who.int/meeting/rc/rc56/rc56_2.htm

TABLE OF CASES

Vinluan v. Doyle, 60 A.D.3d 237 [New York 2d Dept 2009].

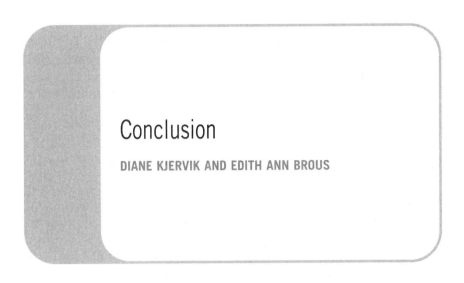

Conclusion

DIANE KJERVIK AND EDITH ANN BROUS

FUTURE ROLES AND OPPORTUNITIES FOR APNs

The future holds rich opportunities for advanced practice nursing (APN) practice, research, education, and policy to evolve together. Just as the law accompanied the change in APN roles over time, at first resisting the change, but gradually embracing it, the law and its ethical counterpart will be part of the increasing independence of APN practice.

Unfolding health care reform approaches will give APNs opportunities to develop more primary, preventive care, hospital, and community-based roles with individuals, families, and communities. The move away from a supervisory model toward a collaborative model of the APN–MD relationship will enhance the development of nursing role and practice.

By embracing the study of law as it affects and is affected by APNs' practice, particularly at the DNP level, APNs are well positioned to make meaningful changes in health policy. Policy leadership is expected at the DNP level, and sophisticated understanding of the law will enhance leadership opportunities.

Drawing on their nursing skills in building trust-based interpersonal relationships, APNs will be well positioned to avoid lawsuits. The APN's honesty and integrity will serve him or her well as he or she develops professional relationships with patients.

As APNs practice across international borders, they will be able to become increasing culturally proficient and will face the challenges of migration laws. Yet, it is clear that with the increasing global economy and the development of international partnerships between universities and health care agencies, APNs will join the international circles of health professionals and agencies to achieve health care and business aspirations.

POTENTIAL LEGAL CHALLENGES TO APN PRACTICE

Although the opportunities are many, the mountains to climb to reach the ambitious goals of APNs are considerable. The number of rules and regulations at state and federal levels result in confusing choices for APNs. Consultation with an attorney will be essential to making decisions about incorporating a practice, engaging in employment and other contractual obligations, using proper billing practices, and building collaborative agreements, to name a few. Where ethically embedded policy choices exist, APNs will be able to work through these gray areas using self-reflection and consultation with other health care professionals, either individually or in groups such as ethics committees. APNs can also use ethical frames of reference, such as virtue ethics, deontology, or care-based ethics to assess patients and choose interventions that fall within the value systems of both patient and APN.

Awareness of the impact of advocacy in certain policies is critical to the overall business health of APN practice. As an example, caps on damage awards in tort reform initiatives have resulted in the unintended consequence of increased complaints about health care professionals to licensure boards. Accordingly, APNs will be well served by purchasing professional liability insurance policies that include licensure defense as a policy benefit. The new apology statutory language may improve APN–patient relationships, but whether this policy will actually result in fewer lawsuits is yet to be examined.

When APNs work through staffing agencies, they must realize that they might be considered the "servant" of both the hospital where they practice and the staffing agency, and might be held liable for actions taken on behalf of both. Their documentation should clearly indicate the type of control both agencies have over the APN's practice.

Challenges remain in the area of labor law, in which APNs might be classified as part of the same collective bargaining group as physicians. APNs prefer separate bargaining groups as more reflective of their employment needs, and have been successful, in some cases, in making this argument. Collaboration with physicians does not mean concerns about wages, working conditions, qualifications, and business practices are the same. Classifying an APN as a supervisor and thus excluding him or her from the bargaining unit is another labor law issue affecting APN practice. For APNs wishing the representation of the union and believing that they are workers who share a community of interest with other nurses, they will need to prepare to work to achieve this goal.

While the challenges to be faced by APNs as their roles evolve are great, in unity, they will achieve their hopes. The Advanced-Practice Registered Nurse consensus statement is an example of the unified vision that provides direction for the future. In spite of a popular president's opposition, the nursing community united to create a nursing research center at the National Institutes of Health. Congress overroode the President's veto and created the National Center (now Institute) of Nursing Research in the mid-1980s. APNs will continue to struggle against such seemingly overwhelming odds to achieve their goals.

APNs have contributed to improvement of public health, and the authors envision that this role will continue to expand. We anticipate that ethical and legal principles will continue to evolve as nursing, particularly in advanced roles, makes its critical contribution to the global community. And an understanding of these principles will remain essential to the education and practice of APNs.

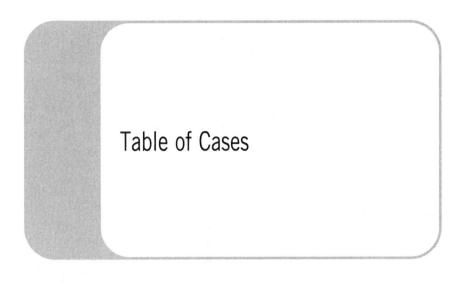

Table of Cases

Central Anesthesia Associates v. Worthy, Castro v. Worthy, Moorehead v. Worthy, Executive Committee of the Baptist Convention v. Worthy, 254 Ga. 728, 333 S.E.2d 829 (1985).
Chico Feminist Women's Health Center v. Butte Glenn Medical Society, 557 F. Supp. 1190 (1983).
Cook v. Worker's Compensation Department, 758 P.2d 854, 306 Or. 134 (1988).
Connecticut Medical Insurance Co. v. Kulikowski, 286 Conn. 1 (2008).
Coombes v. Florio, 450 Mass. 182 (2007).
Corcoran v. Board of Nursing, 197 Or. App. 517 (2005).
Cornfeldt v. Tongen, 262 N.W.2d 684 (1977).
Dalrymple v. George Regional Health System, S.D. Miss. (2009).
Damm v. Axelrod, 148 A.D.2d 974, 539 N.Y.S.2d 210 (1989).
Darling v. Charleston Hospital, 33 Ill.2d 326 (1965).
Devers-Scott v. Office of Prof. Regulation, 918 A.2d 230 (Vt. 2007).
DiFiore v. American Airlines, Inc., 454 Mass. 486 (2009).
Doege v. Sid Peterson Memorial Hospital, 04-04-00570-Cv Tex. App. 4th D. (2005).
Elacqua v. Physicians' Reciprocal Insurers, 21 A.D.3d 702 NY 3d Dept (2005).
Elshoff v. North Carolina Bd. of Nursing, 658 S.E.2d 65 (N.C. App. 3-18-2008).
Ewen v. Baton Rouge General Hospital, 378 So.2d 172 (1979).
Fair Oaks Anesthesia Associates, P.C. v. National Labor Relations Board, 975 F.2d 1068 (4th Cir. September 17, 1992).
Fein v. Permanente Medical Group, 38 Cal.3d 137, 695 P.2d 665, 211 Cal. Rptr. 368 (1985).
Forney v. Memorial Hospital, 543 S.W.2d 705 (1976).
Fortson v. McNamara, 508 So.2d 35 (1987).
Freed v. Geisinger Medical Center, 971 A.2d 1202 Pa. (2009).
Gaines v. Comanche County Medical Hospital, Ok 39 (2006).
Gamble v. United States v. University Anesthesiologists, 648 F. Supp. 438 (1986).
Garrett v. United States, 667 F. Supp. 1147 (1987).
Gehre v. Coleman, 233 Neb. 32, 443 N.W.2d 606 (1989).
Gordon v. Hurlston, 854 So.2d 469 (La. App. 3 Cir. 9/10/03).
Gore v. United States, 229 F. Supp. 547 (1964).
Gershuny v. Martin McFall Messenger Anesthesia Professional Association, 539 So.2d 1131 (1989).
Grover v. Isom, 137 Idaho 770 (2002).
Hammond v. Cty. of Los Angeles, 160 Cal. App. 4th 1579 (2008).
Harris v. Miller, 335 N.C. 379 (1994).
Hospital General Menonita v. NLRB, 393 F.3d 263 (1st Cir. 2004).
Hughes v. St. Paul Fire & Marine, 401 So.2d 448 (1981).
Hyde v. State, 189 Ga. App. 727, 377 S.E.2d 187 (1989).
Hypolite v. Columbia Dauterive Hospital, 968 So.2d 239 La (2007).
Hytko v. Hennessey, 96697 3d Dept (5/7/2009).
In re "Agent Orange" Product Liability Litigation, 689 F. Supp. 1250 (1988). S.2d 813 (1984).
In re Lakatos, 939 A.2d 510 (Vt. 2007).
In the Disciplinary Matter of Greene, 2009 WY 42.
Jones v. Harrisburg Polyclinic Hospital, 496 Pa. 465, 437 A.2d 1134 (1981).
Jones v. Mercy Health Center, Inc., 155 P.3d 9 Ok (2006).

Sweeney v. Athens Regional Medical Center, 709 F. Supp. 1563 (Mar. 1989).

Talmore v. Baptist Hospitals, 09-06-024 Cv Tex. App. 9th Dist. (10/12/2006).

Tarasoff v. Regents of University of California, 17 Cal.3d 425 (1976).

Tempkin v. Lewis-Gale Hospital, Inc., 1989 WL 161163 (W.D.Va.) (1989).

Tesoro v. Alvarez, 13-08-00091-CV Tex. App. 13th Dist. (3/12/2009).

Tuma v. Board of Nursing, 100 Idaho 74 (1979).

Vinluan v. Doyle, 60 A.D.3d 237 [New York 2d Dept 2009].

Vizcaino v. Microsoft Corp., 290 F.3d 1043 (9th Cir. 2002).

Vizcaino v. US Dist. Court for W.D. of Wa, 173 F.3d 713 (9th Cir. 1999).

Vlahos v. Schroeffel, No. 02-CV-0139 (E.D.N.Y. Mar. 6, 2006).

Washington County Mem. Hosp. v. Sidebottom, 7 S.W.3d 542 (Mo.App.E.D. 1999).

Wedgeworth v. Spohn Health, 13-05-446-Cv (Tex. App. [13th Dist.] 4-10-2008).

Whitney v. Day, 100 Mich. App. 707, 300 N.W.2d 380 (1981).

Wicker v. Union County General Hospital, 673 F. Supp. 177 (1987).

Woolbers v. Finley Hospital, 673 N.W.2d 728 Iowa (2003).

Yorston v. Pennell, 397 Pa. 28, 153 A.2d 255 (1959).

Index